Enhancing the health of older people in long-term care

CLINICAL GUIDELINES

Prepared by the Royal Surgical Aid Society-AgeCare,

the British Geriatrics Society and the Research Unit

of the Royal College of Physicians

ROYAL COLLEGE OF PHYSICIANS OF LONDON

1998

ROYAL COLLEGE OF PHYSICIANS OF LONDON
11 St Andrews Place, London NW1 4LE

Registered Charity No 210508

British Cataloguing in Publication Data
A catalogue record for this book is available from the British Library

Copyright © 1998 Royal College of Physicians

ISBN 1 86016 076 X

Designed and typeset by the Publications Unit of the Royal College of Physicians
Printed in Great Britain by Sarum Print Limited, Salisbury, Wiltshire

Contents

Preface by Dr John Wedgwood	v
Acknowledgements	vi

SECTION 1
Introduction	1

SECTION 2
Methods	3

SECTION 3
Challenges for collaboration	4

SECTION 4
Clinical effectiveness and clinical guidelines	10
1. Positive care for people with dementia	10
Clinical guidelines	14
2. Detecting and managing depression	16
Clinical guidelines	19
3. Overcoming disability	21
Clinical guidelines	24
4. Preserving autonomy	26
Clinical guidelines	28
5. Promoting urinary continence	30
Clinical guidelines	32
6. Promoting faecal continence	34
Clinical guidelines	36
7. Optimising medication	38
Clinical guidelines	40
8. Preventing and managing falls	42
Clinical guidelines	44
9. Preventing and managing pressure sores	46
Clinical guidelines	47

SECTION 5
Advice for providers: implementation and outcomes	49

SECTION 6
Advice for commissioners/purchasers 52

SECTION 7
Research and development needs 54

SECTION 8
Conclusion 55

APPENDIX 1
Possible activities 56

APPENDIX 2
Members of the workshops 58

References 61

Further reading 70

Preface

The move in long-term care away from the long stay geriatric hospitals and towards the charitable and private sectors has profoundly altered the balance between hospital and nursing home or residential care. Care in the community has not yet appreciably altered this situation.

Long stay hospital wards, geriatric or psychogeriatric, had a supporting network of monitoring and training facilities, based on teaching and training schools, which set standards for curricula and examinations and undertook traditional audit programmes. Nursing homes could not take these benefits or resources with their patients, so clinical and patient satisfaction audits are not common.

Registration and statutory visits by regulating authorities have mostly been concerned with nursing or residential home facilities, health and safety at work and general patient satisfaction. They have been less concerned with clinical audit, though different authorities vary in this – a variation that itself creates problems.

The CARE scheme for clinical audit proposed and implemented by the Royal College of Physicians in 1992 has an ingenious programme not only to audit but also to monitor and train. The CARE scheme, which has been highly successful, is mainly concerned with physical aspects of care and does not focus on elderly people with predominant dementia. Most nursing homes carry a significant number of elderly people with various degrees of dementia. Some agencies are now developing dedicated homes for the more severely afflicted. RSAS-AgeCare opened its first nursing home with dedicated beds for demented elderly people, the Bradbury Centre, in 1995. RSAS-AgeCare participated in the evaluation project of the CARE scheme and subsequent CARE workshops in Manchester and London.

The Royal Surgical Aid Society is delighted to be asked by the Research Unit of the Royal College of Physicians (RCP) to take an initiative to extend the CARE scheme to cover additional domains (including dementia care) by organising and sponsoring a workshop at the Royal Society of Medicine in 1995. In this way, with representatives of the Royal College of Psychiatrists and other major Royal Colleges and health care organisations, RSAS-AgeCare has with pleasure helped in the preparation of the second edition of this report on high quality long-term care as a basis for an expanded edition of the Royal College of Physicians CARE scheme.

We commend this report and the revised CARE scheme for use in all registered nursing homes and National Health Service continuing care hospital units.

JOHN WEDGWOOD
Chairman, Royal Surgical Aid Society–AgeCare

Acknowledgements

This report would not have been possible without the valuable foundation of its first edition produced by the members of the original workshop.

The Manchester workshop was organised at the Humphrey Booth Institute of Rehabilitation and Gerontology, a collaboration between the Humphrey Booth Trust and the Salford Health Authority, which aims to advance the art and science of the health and social care of older people.

The London workshop was made possible with the help of the Royal Surgical Aid Society–AgeCare (RSAS–AgeCare). RSAS–AgeCare, one of England's longest established charities, seeks new and better ways to care for older infirm people. Its residential and nursing homes have therefore a philosophy of continuous improvement in the provision of high standard long-term care to people who suffer physical or mental infirmity or both.

The Research Unit of the Royal College of Physicians develops and publishes clinical effectiveness materials. It is supported by grants from the Wolfson and Welton Foundations, by other charitable donations and grants, and by a grant from the Department of Health. In addition, the programme of research and development in health care of older people is supported by Private Patients Plan Medical Trust Ltd. This report has been produced and edited independently of any funders.

Introduction

Good health is a key contributor to quality of life amongst older people in long-term care. Access to good health care ranks alongside considerations such as dignity, privacy, independence, choice, rights and fulfilment [Centre for Policy on Ageing 1996]. However, there is still concern about the quality of health care provided [Nolan *et al* 1995b] and the consequences for individuals, families and the nation. The number of older people entering long-term care has continued to grow in the UK since the 1980s. In 1994, £8 bn was spent on providing long-term care for older people [Laing & Buisson 1995]; the debate on long-term financing continues and the quality of care varies. However, there has been insufficient focus on the quality of care, positive approaches to quality improvement and associated cost savings.

This report contains clinical guidelines for enhancing the quality of health care of older people in long-term care. These tackle common clinical challenges that have an obvious link to quality of life. Implementation of the clinical guidelines in this report could transform the health of older people in long-term care. In addition, cost savings would be expected by avoiding errors, duplication and inappropriate care. This report updates two previous publications of the Royal College of Physicians [1992a,b] which covered nine aspects of long-term care (Box 1). It considers wider issues, new evidence and introduces three new domains:

Box 1. The domains of the Royal College of Physicians CARE scheme
- Preserving autonomy
- Promoting urinary continence
- Promoting faecal continence
- Optimising medication
- Managing falls and accidents
- Preventing pressure sores
- Optimising the environment and equipment
- Optimising aids and adaptations
- The medical role in long-term care

Positive care for people with dementia

Detecting and managing depression

Overcoming disability

The report is addressed to all involved and interested in the quality of health care in nursing homes, residential homes and NHS long-term care wards, including residents, relatives, providers (staff and management), purchasers (local authorities, health authorities, fundholding general practitioners, insurers and individuals) and policy makers. Information about this report is being spread widely through a variety of channels and networks to maximise its uptake and impact.

Introduction

To accompany this report, an updated clinical audit scheme, using established quality improvement principles, is being produced. This scheme, like the original *CARE scheme (Continuous Assessment Review and Evaluation)* [Royal College of Physicians 1992c], will provide ready made materials and instructions for each health care domain. It will act as a vehicle for a common approach to quality improvement to be promoted by purchasers, providers, regulators and accreditors of long-term care. Multicentre evaluation of the original CARE scheme has shown it to be useful [Dickinson & Brocklehurst 1997], appropriate and acceptable [Harwood & Ebrahim 1994], and effective [Chambers *et al* 1996].

Definitions

For the purposes of clarity, the following terms are used in this report: *long-term care* refers to care in nursing homes, residential homes and NHS continuing care wards; *carer* refers to lay carers such as family and friends; *care staff* refers to formal carers and staff in long-term care; *resident* refers to patients, residents and clients in long-term care.

Methods

This report was developed using a systematic process that aims to fulfil the requirements of the NHS Executive clinical guidelines appraisal scheme. First, the recommendations of the earlier report [RCP 1992a] were formally evaluated in a multicentre project using the CARE scheme; then the literature was searched for new research findings concerning the original domains. Finally two user-focused interdisciplinary workshops were held in 1995. Following this the report was drafted and developed with the help of workshop participants, external reviewers and consultation.

The workshops focused on users' needs and involved several user groups. The range of other interests represented by the participants was wide and interdisciplinary including clinical psychology, commissioning, creative therapy, health service management, medicine (general practice, psychiatry of old age, geriatric medicine), nursing, occupational therapy, organisational audit, pharmacy, physiotherapy, private and voluntary providers, quality improvement, registration, research, social services and the Department of Health. Each workshop was based on a series of precirculated background papers (Box 2).

The report is based on the background papers, published literature, a check of the Cochrane Library, scrutiny of the draft manual of the King's Fund Organisational Audit for nursing homes, and other information received. A modified Delphi technique [Turoff 1970] was used to develop the document; an original draft was modified with three iterations among workshop participants. This procedure is intended to maximise agreement. The report aims to bring together the best available evidence — the needs of residents and their families, the views of experts and the results of trials and other research. The Royal College of Physicians is committed to the review of published clinical guidelines every 3–6 years, as shown by the production of this report.

Box 2. Background papers of the workshops
- A consumer's view
- Enhancing the role of relatives and residents
- The CARE scheme evaluation project
- Making the CARE scheme work for staff
- Including psycho-social aspects of care
- Expanding the role of recreational activities
- Training for dementia care
- Relationships, behaviour and the environment in dementia care
- The management of depression
- Building care teams

Copies of the background papers can be obtained from the Publications Office of the Royal College of Physicians (price £10.00 to cover copying and postage costs).

SECTION 3

Challenges for collaboration

This chapter discusses some of the major issues raised by residents and their families about the quality of long-term care. It indicates how collaborative solutions involving residents, relatives, staff and others can be developed. Two important underlying themes are choice and the need to discern and respond to personal needs continually.

Entry to long-term care

Transition to long-term care is a very significant move for an individual and for society as a whole. It presents a key opportunity for the assessment of health status, the identification of unresolved health challenges and potential rehabilitation to commence the personalised care planning process. There should be precise roles for the entry assessment but these are inadequately addressed in current entry procedures and the process is not interdisciplinary [Dickinson 1996]. Most older people have mixed feelings about entering residential care. For some people it is a positive choice but for others it may seem like a final loss creating fear and uncertainty [Department of Health 1994]. Fear may be diminished by involving the older people themselves in the decision to enter long-term care, and by maintaining continuity to reduce relocation stress. Another measure that can help reduce fear is the involvement and cooperation of all parties in planning and preparing for the move, and having a key worker on duty when a new resident arrives [Bender *et al* 1996].

Personal needs and care plans

Residents value personal care, good facilities and companionship [Counsel and Care 1992a]. Individual needs are best expressed in personal care plans which can enhance the quality of life of residents especially if they include thorough pre-admission health and social care assessments, biographical information and residents' aspirations. Although a variety of conflicts may arise after admission (Box 3), residents may be reluctant to express discontent with their care. For instance, one study showed a high level of positive response on a Life Satisfaction Index which did not correlate with the researchers' observations [Pearson *et al* 1993]. There is thus a need for care plans to be regularly reviewed and supported with various advocacy approaches.

Box 3. Potential conflicts after admission to long-term care

Tension
- Between residents who are alert but physically disabled and those who are mobile but have dementia

Disappointment
- Lack of social and recreational activity
- Staff seem to have the upper hand
- Poor meals

Frustration
- Inability to express one's feelings about life in the home
- Things promised but not done
- Difficulty in obtaining outside professional care
- Confusion about which staff member to relate to

Death

The mortality rate of people in long-term care is high. Specific guidance on death and dying is to be found in *A better home life* [Centre for Policy on Ageing 1996]. The death of a resident may have strong emotional effects on other residents and staff members. This requires recognition in different ways, and in some cases a memorial service may be appropriate. In any case, concealment of the event should be avoided [Counsel and Care 1995a]. A recent study [Sumaya-Smith 1995] showed that 52% of staff were emotionally affected by the death of a resident. Special consideration must be given to young members of staff who are often required to cope with deep emotional loss without training or counselling.

The relatives' position

Three perspectives of the relative are recognised as being important: their views about care, their role in care and their personal reactions. Relatives are appreciative of the hard work and dedication of staff, often judging the quality of care on the social and emotional care given by staff, as much as on the technical tasks [Duncan & Morgan 1994]. There are also some practical issues that appear to give relatives particular concern when staff are too few or there is lack of training [White 1994]:

- Residents who are not kept clean and have their clothes muddled
- Residents being around for hours with no staff communication
- Confused residents wandering without apparently being noticed
- Residents who cannot move and seem to be neglected

Relatives have to establish a *modus vivendi* with care staff, expressing their views without fear of reprisal and finding their way to continue contributing to the resident's welfare. Good communication between staff, residents and relatives is essential, and this extends to general practitioners, consultants and other professional staff. Many may wish to participate in discussion groups or relatives' committees, and some may want to continue with practical care. Both relatives and residents should be consulted on proposed changes in structure or management in the home. Most relatives feel a great deal of guilt about not doing the caring themselves and, if they have been carers, experience a sense of loss and have to rebuild their own lives [Gladstone 1995]. High levels of depression among family care-givers of older people in long-term care have been reported; the strongest contributing cause is difficulty with the staff [Rosenthal *et al* 1993].

Collaboration and partnership

To tackle these and other issues from a resident's perspective requires a caring partnership between residents, relatives, staff, managers and other interested parties. The clinical guidelines in this report lay foundations for this partnership through a common approach reinforced by the organisational implications that are described along with each guideline. The latter also need to consider and be based on the roles of staff training, teamwork, management, clinical input and quality improvement.

Staff training

There is recurrent concern about the competence of staff, as well as wide recognition that they carry out difficult and demanding work, often with inadequate numbers. These issues, together with frequently changing staff, the low priority given to training and the general low regard in which work among older people is held, form a vicious circle [Dimond 1986; Kayser-Jones 1990; Gilloran et al 1993]. Residents can become depersonalised 'work objects' with too much task orientation and low levels of work interest and satisfaction [Wells 1980; Reed & Bond 1991; Waters 1994]. Training can have far reaching tangible and intangible benefits (Box 4). Staff need a knowledge base (at least normal ageing and the common health challenges of old age) and appropriate attitudes. They should have communication skills and be good at working with families [Chartock et al 1988; Webber 1991; Jones et al 1992; Kihlgren et al 1993]. The physical and emotional demands of caring can lead to stress among staff [Baillon et al 1996], so consideration of their needs is essential to promote high quality care. For example, the ability to remain relaxed and smiling when carrying out care can be important in deflecting behavioural crises [Burgener & Barton 1991; Burgener et al 1992]. This involves training and managing staff with positive feedback on their performance [Murphy 1992; Alfredson & Annerstedt 1994; Nystrom & Segerston 1994; Gilloran et al 1995], and requires skill, commitment, personal involvement, imagination and creativity [Scott 1995]. Local joint training groups for staff, volunteers and carers working in residential, day care, domiciliary, sheltered housing and other care settings may be useful.

> **Box 4. Some benefits of training**
>
> **Improvement in staff motivation**
> - Enhanced perception of work in long-term care [Feldt & Ryden 1992]
> - Increased staff morale, self confidence and job satisfaction [Lardner & Nicholson 1990; Nolan 1992; Nolan & Walker 1993]
>
> **Improvement in care**
> - Reduction in sedation [Rovner et al 1996]
> - Environmental changes [Nolan 1992]
> - Greater autonomy and independence of residents [Nolan 1992; Nolan & Walker 1993]
> - More participation and interaction between staff and residents [Kihlgren et al 1993; Alfredson & Annerstedt 1994; Miller 1995]
> - Innovations in care [Nolan et al 1995b]

The organisational setting for training is vital, as articulated in the national training accreditation scheme Investors in People. If training is to be effective, staff must see the need for it and believe it will result in beneficial change [Palmer 1995]. Staff should be encouraged to acquire specialist skills, become trainers and by raising the expectations for development amongst all care staff [Nolan 1992; Nolan & Walker 1993; Nolan et al 1995a]. Staff should also be involved in the design, content and delivery of the training programme which should be given priority by management. Training should be based on modern principles of adult learning [Alfredson & Annerstedt 1994; Gilloran et al 1995]. There are natural links between training, quality improvement and management as discussed below [Kitwood & Woods 1996]. At a practical level, use of the CARE scheme may assist in gaining National Vocational Qualifications. Teaching nursing homes have wide acceptance in medical training in the USA [Katz et al 1995]. Medical schools and faculties of nursing in the UK could explore this approach of working with nursing homes as an appropriate training resource for students and trainees. Both undergraduate and postgraduate training are relevant.

Teamwork

Overall, many professional disciplines may have an input to the health care of older people (Box 5), though the day to day delivery of long-term care rests mainly with nurses and care assistants. The team approach to the health care of older people is now accepted and this should be reflected in long-term care [Department of Health 1996a, 1997]. In organisational terms, a team should be a group of workers who collaborate together with agreed aims, goals and objectives, working in a formalised way with a clear understanding of each other's roles and expectations. Difficulties in extending the team structure include lack of common metaphors, models, theories and vocabularies among professionals concerned [Jones et al 1992]. Organisation of work should entail networking, with most of the other disciplines (Box 5) called in, if accessible, as and when required.

Box 5. Professional disciplines involved in long-term care (alphabetical order)
- Chaplaincy
- Chiropody
- Clinical psychology
- Counselling
- Dietetics
- Management
- Medicine (primary care, geriatric medicine, psychiatry of old age etc)
- Nursing (including continence promotion, tissue viability etc)
- Occupational therapy
- Pharmacology
- Physiotherapy
- Social work
- Speech and language therapy

Quality improvement

In the past there has been heavy reliance on inspection alone to safeguard the quality of long-term care. To enhance health care in long-term care there is a strong need and emphasis for a complementary quality improvement approach, which is a management responsibility since it interfaces with other issues such as the use of resources, general management style and staff training. Such an approach is matched by the introduction of clinical audit in the NHS. The CARE scheme should therefore be adopted as the quality improvement system in long-term care since it meets the principles of quality improvement, allows staff to examine the quality of their work, and provides a framework for staff and management to work together to achieve common quality goals. National comparative audit using the CARE scheme may allow benchmarking. An added benefit of this scheme is its potential for accreditation through schemes such as the King's Fund Organisational Audit. There are no real incentives, other than intrinsic factors, for individual long-term care facilities to take steps to improve the quality of health care for their residents. However, through benchmarking and accreditation, individual residents and their families could be reassured about receiving the best care, and national benefits in

Challenges for collaboration

the health of the older population would be demonstrated. Leadership and expertise are required to promote quality improvement in health care, preferably through clinical audit.

Management

Management style is important in delivering high quality long-term care. Some would argue that the complexity of delivering good personalised care demands some of the very best management skills. Managers should be primarily concerned with how they can best support their staff in meeting the needs of residents. This can be met with an appropriate management style that values and trains staff, nurtures teamwork and promotes quality improvement to empower staff as described. The potentially stressful nature of long-term care nursing has been acknowledged [Hallberg & Norberg 1995]. There is a strong relationship between job satisfaction and quality of care provided [Robertson et al 1995].

Clinical input

In the future there is likely to be increasing emphasis on clinical input in achieving high quality health care in long-term care. At present significant challenges exist in relation to all the disciplines.

- *Primary care*. The role of the general practitioner (GP) is often debated and work patterns have been described as chaotic [Bowman 1996]. At present it is up to most residents to retain their own GPs. This may conflict with the feasibility of having multiple visiting GPs, the possible classification of the medical care of highly dependent patients in the community as a 'non-core' activity, and the need for access to committed expertise. There is a need for the facility and medical practitioners to have the same philosophy and values of care, and the opportunity to talk about aspects of care ranging from end of life decisions to daily life in the home.

- *Specialist care*. Geriatricians and old age psychiatrists are key specialist expertise sources with experience of teamwork. In NHS continuing care wards this is reasonably straightforward because each patient is in the care of a consultant. In other long-term care settings, arrangements for liaison are not universal. Geriatricians have a strategic role as 'the torch bearers for improving the care of these most vulnerable of patients' [Webster 1994], but models of liaison are underdeveloped. With good leadership, consultants are instrumental in achieving good outcomes [Kayser-Jones 1991]. However, wide variation in the level of involvement and commitment among medical directors has been demonstrated [Elon 1993].

- *Nurses*. They are likely to have an increasingly prominent role in long-term care. A large multicentre study in the United States showed that specialist nurses were as good as family physicians according to a range of measures such as level of disability, use of medication, management of tracer conditions (such as new urinary incontinence) and use of emergency and hospital services [Kane et al 1991].

- *Therapists*. Physiotherapists, occupational therapists, activities organisers and others have an important role in long-term care, particularly in overcoming disability and handicap. Effective involvement with residents and good collaboration with other staff are vital in carrying out this role.

- *Costs.* There may be a conflict between quality care and the fees offered to providers. This report emphasises that sufficient staff with appropriate skills are instrumental in providing high quality care. But it does not necessarily mean that quality care is always costly, or that lack of quality is due to poor quality staff. Substandard management, staff training and staff support may also be reasons.

SECTION 4

Clinical effectiveness and clinical guidelines

This chapter introduces three health care domains new to this report — **positive care for people with dementia**, **detecting and managing depression** and **overcoming disability** — and updates previous domains. Evidence is given in a common format which examines in turn why the domain needs to be addressed (*Rationale*), the present quality of care (*Quality of care*) and what should be done to achieve high quality care (*Requirements*). Following this review of clinical effectiveness, clinical guidelines for each domain are represented in a standard layout. These guidelines are aimed at enhancing the quality of care and hence the outcomes of care. They are based on the perspectives of residents and care staff, expert opinion and best available evidence. Their organisational implications offer benefits to all stakeholders in long-term care and provide a sound approach to high quality services for people in long-term care. The clinical guidelines for each domain are presented for easy photocopying by the staff of a facility.

1. Positive care for people with dementia (new domain)

RATIONALE

Three-quarters of residents in long-term care have dementia [Rovner *et al* 1990; Schneider *et al* 1997] and they should receive a standard of care comparable to that received by those without dementia. The new culture of dementia care presents positive and optimistic approaches in dementia care, thereby retaining many positive and fulfilling experiences for dementia sufferers and providing rewarding experiences for their carers. Traditional ways of working therefore need to be challenged and radically changed [Counsel and Care 1996a]. There are major challenges in providing an appropriate environment, ensuring positive staff attitudes and in the suitable management of 'challenging' behaviours (eg wandering, aggression, night-time disturbance, shouting, incontinence). From an economic point of view there is a need for high quality care to avoid costly complications and adverse events. Dementia is very difficult and bewildering for relatives, who need help and cooperation from staff to uplift their morale [Stephens *et al* 1991; Ritchie & Ledésert 1992]. Further, disparities in perceptions of mental disorders across disciplines suggest a need for incorporation of mental health expertise in long term settings [Podgorski *et al* 1996].

QUALITY OF CARE

Shortcomings in the quality of dementia care can result in aimless care [Evers 1991] and failure to meet the needs of residents. At worst the resident is ignored as a person and physical and drug restraint are used. Staff may concentrate on the tasks in hand rather than the person, because the work is physically and emotionally exhausting. One study found that 50% of staff could not see any meaning in the lives of residents with dementia [Kuremyr *et al* 1994].

REQUIREMENTS

There are considerable difficulties in carrying out randomised controlled trials of care for people with dementia; the basis for high quality care therefore rests mainly on observational and developmental work.

1. Positive care for people with dementia

- *General.* The philosophy should aim at high levels of well-being, including people with severe dementia, by adopting a positive approach that highlights residual strengths and aspects capable of amelioration [Kitwood 1993]. This can be supported by personalised care plans that recognise all residents as individuals with a wide variety of life experiences and influences and differing in needs and abilities [Guaita *et al* 1995]. Collaboration with relatives should be the norm, to assist the formation of relationships between staff and residents and the promotion of stimulating activity [Nolan 1992]. Findings from a recent study indicate that families/carers were involved in the review of care plans, which were in general reviewed annually. However, there was variability in the policy and practice for review, and evidence of multidisciplinary care planning appeared limited [Moriarty & Webb 1997].

- *Identification and diagnosis of cognitive impairment.* People with dementia need to be clearly diagnosed as such and have their level of cognitive functioning assessed and reviewed regularly using recognised methods. Care needs and the occurrence of challenging behaviour are often greater in the presence of cognitive impairment [Aronson *et al* 1993], whether related to delirium (also known as acute confusional state) or a dementia syndrome (often due to Alzheimer's disease). These can and should be distinguished using an approach such as the Confusion Assessment Method [Inouye *et al* 1990].

- *Cause.* The cause of dementia should be diagnosed for an understanding of its course and prognosis.

- *Preventing and stopping challenging behaviours.* The Brief Agitation Rating scale is a checklist for a variety of behaviours [Finkel *et al* 1993]. Possible sources (Box 6) of challenging behaviours can be identified which suggest preventive measures [Nelson 1995]. Of these, depression and restraint merit special attention. The Alzheimer's Disease Society produces a series of advice sheets which should be available to staff concerning the management of inappropriate behaviours.

- *Restraint.* Restraint by drugs or any other means should be avoided [Counsel and Care 1992b, 1993a]. Tranquillisers and sedatives are the drugs most commonly used in restraint; although they have a limited role, in small doses, for specific purposes such as the treatment of agitation, hyperactivity, hallucination or hostility [Sunderland & Silver 1988], many homes successfully care for residents without them. A high prevalence of 'inappropriate' neuroleptic prescribing has been reported [McGrath & Jackson 1996]. Caution should be exercised with neuroleptics, and medication should be thoroughly reviewed regularly. Reverting to locked doors, the use of tagging and internal video monitoring is controversial; whilst 'a degree of surveillance and protection is implicit, greater clarity is required in specifying what sort of restraint is permissible' [Counsel and Care 1993b, 1996b].

- *Environment.* This should be safe, secure, prosthetic, quiet, small and well designed. Good lighting and appropriate orientation aids, such as careful signposting and clocks, are important. Accurate, succinct information for residents should be provided, with care to avoid information overload.

Clinical effectiveness and clinical guidelines

- *Activity*. This can include music, exercise, crafts, relaxation, reminiscence, religious observance, word games and food preparation. Minimisation of the use of psychotropic drugs to diminish behaviour problems and the consequent use of restraints must also be considered [Rovner *et al* 1996]. The effect of exercise in diminishing behaviour problems has been reviewed [Beck *et al* 1992].

- *Access to specialist advice*. Routes of referral and liaison with the local team for the psychiatry of old age should be established.

Box 6. The Brief Agitation Rating scale checklist of challenging behaviours
- ❏ Hitting
- ❏ Grabbing
- ❏ Pushing
- ❏ Pacing or aimless wandering
- ❏ Performing repetitious mannerisms
- ❏ Restlessness
- ❏ Screaming
- ❏ Repetitive sentences or questions
- ❏ Strange noises
- ❏ Complaining

Sources

Internal

Factors worsening confusion (eg depression, acute confusion, medication)

Physical factors and needs (eg disability, discomfort, pain, loss of senses, loss of speech)

Previous personality

Ideas that are out of touch with reality [Kitwood & Bredin 1992a,b]

Emotions (eg anger, apathy, fear, sorrow, loneliness)

Interactions

Poor communication

Negative behaviour of staff and other residents which can promote a cycle of discouragement and depersonalisation

Misinterpretation of events or activities of others as threats

Disputes, including those about possessions

External environment

Restraint by medication or physical means

Lack of clues and cues (eg in toilet)

Overstimulation by distracting inputs

1. Positive care for people with dementia

- *Depression.* The identification and treatment of associated depression should constantly be borne in mind (see *Detecting and managing depression* section).

A positive approach to the care of people with dementia has also been developed in Special Care Units in nursing homes in the United States [Berg et al 1991]. The main components (summarised in Box 7) reflect closely the principles stated above.

Box 7. Management modalities for special care units [Berg et al 1991]

Physical environment
- ❑ Reduction of noxious stimuli (eg noise, glare, crowding)
- ❑ Provision of safe wandering
- ❑ Access to outdoors
- ❑ Clues to finding one's way
- ❑ Visual, tactile, musical and other sensory stimulation

Staff approaches to care
- ❑ Individualised care planning and provision
- ❑ A team approach to care, with consistent staffing
- ❑ Behaviour modification
- ❑ Minimisation of physical and pharmacological restraints
- ❑ Emphasis on the patients' dignity

Therapeutic programmes
- ❑ Approaches and activities appropriate for residents' cognitive and functional status
- ❑ Focus on residents' strengths and familiar activities such as religious, cultural and ethnic rituals
- ❑ Group occupational, physical and activity therapy programmes such as cooking, gardening, dancing, exercise, sensory stimulation
- ❑ One-to-one activities such as ball throwing, review of photo albums, hand massage

Involvement of families
- ❑ Encouragement of family participation in activities and care
- ❑ Provision of information and support groups

Clinical effectiveness and clinical guidelines

CARE GUIDELINE

ASSESSMENT

All residents should have a documented assessment on entry, and regularly thereafter, covering:

- Assessment of cognitive function using a recognised scale (such as the Abbreviated Mental Test)
- Clear diagnosis of the cause(s) of cognitive impairment, with specialist assistance if necessary
- For those with dementia, assessment to understand and prevent challenging behaviour
- A detailed account of the person's life history, including important experiences and relationships, to encourage a holistic approach to the person

CARE PLAN

All residents with dementia should have a personalised care plan implemented that covers:

- The goals of care and the roles of different staff members
- Specific aspects of care:
    - Development of relationships with staff
    - Avoidance of restraint and sedation
    - Preventing and managing challenging behaviour (eg wandering)
    - Surveillance for depression
    - 'Purposeful activities'
- Regular review of the implementation and effectiveness of the plan with relatives
- Regular review for referral to a specialist old age psychiatry team if required

ENVIRONMENT

All residents with dementia should experience an appropriate enabling environment, to include:

- Labelling and signing of toilets, bedroom, dining room
- Good lighting
- Freedom from extraneous noise
- Home-like settings
- Safe corridors and doors, with appropriate decorative schemes and clear signposting

SPECIALIST ACCESS

All residents with dementia should have access to the advice of the local old age psychiatry team.

INFORMATION, INVOLVEMENT AND SATISFACTION

The relatives of all residents with dementia should:

- Have clearly communicated information about the diagnosis and their part in the care plan
- Be regularly consulted about the policy, plans, staff development and quality improvement for *positive care for people with dementia*
- Be satisfied with care in relation to dementia

1. Positive care for people with dementia

ORGANISATIONAL IMPLICATIONS

COMMITMENT

All long-term care facilities should show commitment to *positive care for people with dementia* by:

- Having a policy as described below
- Effectively communicating this to all staff on joining, and at regular intervals
- Providing the required resources to put the policy into action
- Supporting the policy by staff development and quality improvement

POLICY AND PLANNING

All long-term care facilities should have a written agreed policy to implement the care guidelines that includes:

- A philosophy of *positive care for people with dementia*
- The role of different staff members and others in working as a team
- The approach to assessment
- The procedure for devising and implementing a personalised care plan, including detailed contents, review mechanism and onward referral system
- Relevant aspects of the environment
- Agreements on access to specialists
- The provision of information to and involvement of relatives as well as a commitment to satisfaction

STAFF DEVELOPMENT

All long-term care facilities should support the policy by regular staff development activities that:

- Are structured, organised and comprehensive
- Are relevant to all levels of staff
- Cover the range of required knowledge, attitudes, skills and roles
- Are developed, implemented and evaluated using principles of adult learning
- Follow best practice in clinical supervision, encouraging reflective practice

QUALITY IMPROVEMENT

All long-term care facilities should carry out quality improvement activities, such as clinical audit, to achieve high standards of *positive care for people with dementia*.

2. Detecting and managing depression *(new domain)*

RATIONALE

Many older people feel depressed for a variety of reasons and for varying lengths of time, but depression is not inevitable [Counsel and Care 1995b]. Depression is common among long-term care residents, affecting up to 50% [Rovner *et al* 1990; Weyerer *et al* 1995; Age Concern 1996]. It often remains undetected or neglected although it increases the likelihood of death [Rovner *et al* 1991]. Broadly there are two types of depression [Parker & Hadzi-Pavlovic 1993]:

- *'Dimensional' depression* presents with many depressive symptoms, though social function is preserved, and improves immediately within the first two weeks of admission [Engle & Graney Marshal 1993]. It is found in 30–60% of residents at any time, with lower rates in long-term residents [Mann *et al* 1984].

- *'Categorical' depression* presents with clear symptoms (eg low mood and self esteem, altered sleep pattern, appetite and weight loss, regular daily variation in mood, constipation, suicidal or psychotic ideas) that predict response to antidepressant treatment. It has a prevalence of 20% in long-term care [Ames 1993].

Since the two types of depression overlap, distinction is difficult.

QUALITY OF CARE

The present quality of care for people with depression appears to be inadequate, and recognition rates in long-term care are low [Kivela *et al* 1986]. Possible reasons are shown in Box 8. In a recent study, few general practitioners (6%) had a formal system to identify depression in homes, and most formal systems (85%) relied on nurses to detect it [Age Concern 1996]. Work in the USA has shown that depression in nursing home residents is inadequately and inappropriately treated [Heston *et al* 1992].

Box 8. Reasons for the low rate of recognition of depression

- ❏ The importance of recognising depression may not be appreciated
- ❏ Significant changes in the residents may not be noticed, especially if staff turnover is high or handover procedures are poor or non-existent
- ❏ Time to observe and talk to residents may be insufficient
- ❏ Depression is hard to detect in people with dementia
- ❏ Staff may be poorly trained in detection of psychiatric problems [Godlove *et al* 1980]
- ❏ The GP may not be willing to assess and treat or refer the patient [Weyerer *et al* 1995]

2. Detecting and managing depression

REQUIREMENTS

The recognition and management of depression is vital; evidence of effectiveness is presented as follows.

- *General*. Since depression causes much suffering it is important that it be recognised, treated and prevented, along the promotional lines of the national Defeat Depression campaign [Royal College of Psychiatrists 1996].

- *Recognition*. This depends on specific observation of symptoms and signs [Chester & Smith 1995]. Important predictors of depression are pre-existing depressive illness, physical musculoskeletal symptoms, and lack of visits from friends and relatives [Weyerer *et al* 1995]. Staff should be aware that some types of unusual behaviour (eg tearing or removing clothes, eating faeces, grovelling on the floor, screaming) [Friedman *et al* 1992] are particularly suggestive of depression. Among residents with dementia, special attention should be paid to weight loss [Morley & Kraenzie 1994], appetite change, increased agitation and restlessness (especially when diurnal).

- *Assessment of mood*. The Geriatric Depression Scale has been recommended as a standard scale for detecting depression [RCP 1992b], with the shorter version more convenient in use [Hermann *et al* 1996]. The performance of the scale is improved with previous screening for cognitive impairment [McGivney *et al* 1994]. It has a place in assessment for and on entry, and comparisons can be made with previous assessments. Other measures, such as the card based system BASDEC, are also available [Gerety *et al* 1994; McGivney *et al* 1994].

- *Primary management and the environment*. The initial management of depression is summarised in Box 9. Close, warm interaction between staff and residents is important, promoted through good listening skills, physical contact and positive, welcoming spontaneous gestures [Nagel *et al* 1988; Buschmann & Hollingur 1994]. Residents need social stimulation and a recreation programme will help (Appendix 1 shows a range of possible activities). Depression just before death, and the extent to which rapid treatment should be initiated, pose difficult problems with no definite answer [Simon 1989; McCue 1995].

> **Box 9. Initial care for depression**
>
> **Assessment**
> - Make a thorough assessment of biological, social and psychological aspects of the depression
> - Institute a care plan taking all these into account
> - Check for remediable problems (eg anaemia, heart failure, painful arthritis, depressant drugs such as haloperidol, hypo- or hyper-thyroidism)
>
> **Management**
> - Encourage talking about feelings
> - Encourage activities to lift mood (eg trips, visitors, exercise)
> - Use antidepressants if biological symptoms become prominent
>
> **Review**
> - Ensure adequate dose and duration of antidepressant treatment
> - Be vigilant for suicidal ideas and biological symptoms (eg weight loss, poor fluid intake)
> - Refer for specialist management if suicidal, or antidepressants fail, or significantly depressed state lasts more than 2 months

Clinical effectiveness and clinical guidelines

- *Specialist management.* Results of a randomised controlled trial in a community setting have shown that an individual package of care formulated by a community psychogeriatric team is more effective (odds ratio = 9.0 (confidence interval 2.0–41.5)) in treating depression than normal general practitioner care [Banerjee *et al* 1996]. The package of care included any combination of physical interventions (drugs, physical review), psychological interventions (eg bereavement counselling, family work) and social interventions (eg referral to a day centre, benefit check). However, day hospital and inpatient treatment may be required for suicidal patients and those with especially severe or persistent depressive symptoms. In the case of severe physical illness (eg cancer, arthritis, severe heart failure) an aggressive approach to treatment may not only relieve the depression but also improve the symptoms of the underlying illness [Harnett 1994].

2. Detecting and managing depression

CARE GUIDELINE

ASSESSMENT

All residents should have a documented assessment on entry, and regularly thereafter, that covers:

- Assessment of mood using a recognised scale (such as the Geriatric Depression Scale)
- A clear diagnosis of the cause of low mood, made with the help of a specialist if necessary
- Identification of opportunities to prevent depression, including a review of medication

CARE PLAN

All residents with depression should have an implemented personalised care plan that covers:

- The goals of care and the roles of different staff members
- Specific aspects of care:
    - Social interaction and exercise
    - Antidepressant drug treatment
    - Cognitive therapy
    - Surveillance for weight loss and suicidal ideas/intention
- Regular review of the implementation and effectiveness of the plan in improving mood
- Regular review of the need for onward referral to a specialist old age psychiatry team if unresponsive to a therapeutic regime for 4 weeks

SPECIALIST ACCESS

All residents with depression should have access to the expert advice of the old age psychiatry team and health care of older people team.

ENVIRONMENT

All residents with depression should experience an appropriate supportive environment including:

- Access to recreational activities

INFORMATION, INVOLVEMENT AND SATISFACTION

All residents with depression and their relatives should:

- Have clearly communicated information about the diagnosis and their involvement in the care plan
- Be regularly consulted about the policy, plans, staff development and quality improvement for *detecting and managing depression*
- Be satisfied with care in relation to depression

Clinical effectiveness and clinical guidelines

ORGANISATIONAL IMPLICATIONS

COMMITMENT

All long-term care facilities should show commitment to *detecting and managing depression* by:

- Having a policy as described below
- Effectively communicating this to all staff on joining, and at regular intervals
- Providing the required resources to put the policy into action
- Supporting the policy by staff development and quality improvement

POLICY AND PLANNING

All long-term care facilities should have a written agreed policy to implement the care guidelines that includes:

- A philosophy of *detecting and managing depression*
- The role of different staff members and others in working as a team
- The approach to assessment
- The procedure for devising and implementing a personalised care plan, including detailed contents, review mechanism and onward referral system
- Relevant aspects of the environment
- Agreements on access to specialists
- The provision of information to and involvement of residents and relatives, as well as a commitment to satisfaction

STAFF DEVELOPMENT

All long-term care facilities should support the policy by regular staff development activities that:

- Are structured, organised and comprehensive
- Are relevant to all levels of staff
- Cover the range of required knowledge, attitudes, skills and roles
- Are developed, implemented and evaluated using principles of adult learning

QUALITY IMPROVEMENT

All long-term care facilities should carry out quality improvement activities, such as clinical audit, to achieve high standards in *detecting and managing depression*.

3. Overcoming disability *(new domain)*

RATIONALE

This new section expands and builds on two previous domains of the CARE scheme [RCP 1992c] (***Environment and equipment*** and ***Aids and adaptations***) and focuses on the need to address disability in long-term care from a therapeutic perspective. Overcoming disability so as to minimise handicap is profoundly important for individuals, long-term care facilities and the health of the population. Even small improvements in the functioning of older people may lead to benefits in quality of life and in the quality and costs of care. The importance of life free of disability has been recognised by the EQUAL initiative of the Office of Science and Technology. Numerous surveys have shown the high level of disability in long-term care residents which is thought to be increasing. This section concentrates on primary activities of daily living (apart from using the toilet which is covered in another section) (Box 10), special senses and communication. However, the great importance of secondary activities of daily living (eg cooking, cleaning, shopping) is also acknowledged. Several factors contributing to overcoming disability are considered: recognition of disability, the management of underlying health problems, the role of rehabilitation, the use of personal aids and adaptations, and the role of the environment.

> **Box 10. Primary activities of daily living (ADL)**
> - Mobility
> - Transfers (eg from bed to chair and back)
> - Using the toilet
> - Grooming
> - Bathing
> - Getting dressed
> - Feeding

QUALITY OF CARE

Evidence about how the quality of care contributes to overcoming disability is deficient. Assessment at entry misses opportunities for the management of disability, partly because it has insufficient input from the range of disciplines required [Dickinson 1996]. Common disabilities are not recognised; for example, difficulties with sight and hearing often go undetected. A recent survey disclosed unrecognised significant refractive errors in about a third of residents [Sturgess *et al* 1994]. Similarly, screening for hearing impairment is haphazard: 70% of residents had significant hearing impairment, 47% wanted further help (which was not offered) and fewer than 10% of residents owned and used a hearing aid [Tolson & McIntosh 1992]. Little is known about the specific quality of management of health problems; potential for improvement is discussed for each of the domains in this report. Rehabilitation has not been a feature of long-term care since few people leave long-term care. Many residents rely on aids and equipment but there is very little systematic information about their appropriateness and maintenance. The use of personal aids and adaptations is probably suboptimal, not least because of the low involvement of therapists in long-term care.

Clinical effectiveness and clinical guidelines

REQUIREMENTS

Much of the knowledge based approach to disability depends on sound experience since systematic research is scant.

- *General.* The facility should foster a constructive approach focused on minimising disability and handicap. There are three established principles for effective rehabilitation: interdisciplinary input, teamwork and a goal orientated approach.

- *Recognising disability.* This is needed to plan therapeutic approaches to care, and understand the benefits of prosthetic interventions (such as aids). This is particularly important on entry to long-term care, otherwise remediable disabilities may be missed for ever. There is growing evidence that comprehensive assessment of older people is worthwhile in hospital settings [Stuck *et al* 1993]; this may apply in long-term care, giving the comprehensive entry assessments a scientific basis. The Barthel ADL Index has been recommended as a means of assessing disability in a standard format and is now commonly used. Other measures such as Functional Independence (FIM) [State University of New York 1993], Lambeth Disability Screening Questionnaire (for sensory handicaps) and the Minimum Dataset/Resident Assessment Instrument for a comprehensive assessment [Morris *et al* 1990] might also be useful.

- *Management of underlying health problems.* It is crucial that any underlying health problem be identified. Virtually any health problem may result in disability and may be amenable to medical treatment. Common examples include arthritis, heart failure, Parkinson's disease, hypothyroidism, foot problems and sensory difficulties. Pain can threaten quality of life so it should be assessed and treated appropriately.

- *Rehabilitation.* The care plan should be used to plan for rehabilitation and should include the role of different disciplines and negotiated goals. Therapists can work with staff, particularly in handling and seating residents properly. Consideration of the environment in long-term care is often limited to justifiable interest in homeliness and architectural qualities. However, the environment also has a key role in promoting independence (Box 11). An active and systematic approach to sensory impairment can do much to minimise the disabling effects of sight and hearing loss [DoH 1995]. Rehabilitation may include a wide range of interventions. These should focus on balance, strength, daily living skills, perceptual problems and the use of many existing aids for tackling difficulties in the primary activities of daily living.

- *Environment.* The environment can have a profound effect on disability, though there are few trials to substantiate this. There is a general need for suitable adjustable chairs and appropriate carpeting, handrails, gradients etc. The specific role of the environment is discussed under each domain.

Few long-term care facilities will possess all the necessary knowledge and resources for the best management of disability. This implies the need to establish relationships with local specialists in the hospital and primary care team, and access to the required range of equipment.

3. Overcoming disability

Box 11. Features of aids, adaptations and environment that can help in overcoming disability

Mobility

- Wheelchair: design important, ownership preferable, maintenance vital for tyre inflation, foot rests, seat cushion, brakes
- Walking stick: check height, ferule, correct use
- Walking frame: check size, technique, handles, attachments

Transfers

- Chairs: range of different heights to suit different needs; appropriate seating can increase social interaction [Davies & Snaith 1980]
- Beds: correct height, firmness to suit different needs

Toilet aids

- Includes raised seats, rails, flooring, paper dispenser

Bathing

- Grab rails, bath board, flooring, specialist baths and showers

Getting dressed

- Dressing aids
- Clothing adaptations

Washing and grooming

- Adapted taps
- Wheelchair access

Eating

- Adapted cutlery and crockery

Special senses and communication

- Audio-cassettes are used regularly by a majority of blind people; the nationwide audio-cassette service is highly commended [Marsland *et al* 1994]
- Staff training in communication and guiding skills for work with visually impaired and hearing impaired people
- Spectacles: cleanliness, fit, adjustment
- Access to large print and talking books
- Practical aspects of hearing aids (eg leads, batteries), and limitations on their use

Clinical effectiveness and clinical guidelines

CARE GUIDELINE

ASSESSMENT

All residents should have a documented assessment on entry, and regularly thereafter, including a record of when new health problems arise, and covering:

- Assessment of disability using a recognised scale (such as the Barthel ADL Index)
- A clear diagnosis by a specialist of the underlying health problems causing disability
- Identification of opportunities to promote independence

CARE PLAN

All residents with significant disability should have an implemented personalised care plan that covers:

- The goals of care, the roles of different staff members and teamwork in care
- Specific aspects of care:
    - Management of underlying health problems
    - Scope for further rehabilitation
    - Aids and adaptations
    - Surveillance for worsening disability
- Regular review of the implementation and effectiveness of the plan
- Regular review of the need for onward referral to a specialist

ENVIRONMENT

All residents with significant disability should experience an appropriate environment, to include:

- For mobility: sufficiently wide corridors, ramps, handrails, floor coverings, wheelchair accessibility
- For transfers: bed and chairs of appropriate height
- In the toilet: raised toilet seat, grab rails
- Bathing and washing: bathroom adaptations
- Special senses: appropriate lighting and noise levels

SPECIALIST ACCESS

All residents with significant disability should have access to the specialist team in the health care of older people, community therapists and other local experts.

INFORMATION, INVOLVEMENT AND SATISFACTION

All residents with significant disability and their relatives should:

- Have clearly communicated information and involvement in the care plan
- Be regularly consulted about the policy, plans, staff development and quality improvement for *overcoming disability*
- Be satisfied with care in relation to disability

3. Overcoming disability

ORGANISATIONAL IMPLICATIONS

COMMITMENT

All long-term care facilities should show commitment to *overcoming disability* by:

- Having a policy as described below
- Effectively communicating this to all staff on joining, and at regular intervals
- Providing the required resources to put the policy into action
- Supporting the policy by staff development and quality improvement

POLICY AND PLANNING

All long-term care facilities should have a written agreed policy to implement these care guidelines that includes:

- A philosophy for *overcoming disability*
- The role of different staff members and others in working as a team
- The approach to assessment
- The procedure for devising and implementing a personalised care plan, including detailed contents, review mechanism and onward referral system
- Relevant aspects of the environment
- Agreements on access to specialists
- The provision of information to and involvement of residents and relatives, as well as a commitment to satisfaction

STAFF DEVELOPMENT

All long-term care facilities should support the policy through regular staff development activities that:

- Are structured, organised and comprehensive
- Are relevant to all levels of staff
- Cover the range of required knowledge, attitudes, skills and roles
- Are developed, implemented and evaluated using principles of adult learning

QUALITY IMPROVEMENT

All long-term care facilities should carry out quality improvement activities, such as clinical audit, to achieve high standards in *overcoming disability*.

The following sections update the health care domains covered in the report *High quality long-term care for elderly people* [RCP 1992a] and the *CARE scheme* [RCP 1992c], and contain new evidence concerning the effectiveness and quality of care.

4. Preserving autonomy *(updated)*

RATIONALE

Autonomy is central to long-term care but is often threatened. Goffman [1961] drew attention to life in isolation from general social life where staff tend to feel superior and righteous while inmates feel weak, inferior, blameworthy and guilty [Clark & Bowling 1990]. These attitudes were exemplified by deprivation of personal possessions and clothing, intrusion on privacy, demeaning practices and 'batch living' — all residents being treated alike and doing the same thing at the same time. Similar effects in British long-term care institutions are graphically described in *The last refuge* [Townsend 1962].

QUALITY OF CARE

Evidence shows that approaches to the preservation of autonomy are still inadequate. In a study of long-term care in a hospital ward and two NHS nursing homes, lucid patients' requests were totally ignored by staff in 32% of observation sessions in the ward compared with 18% and 8% in the nursing homes [Clark & Bowling 1990]. Studies have shown that nursing staff interactions with residents in long-term care are superficial, routinised and related to tasks [Armstron-Esther *et al* 1994; Hewison 1995]. This may be due to the power barrier between staff and resident [Hewison 1995]. In a recent large multicentre audit study, approaches to preserving autonomy were incomplete [Brocklehurst & Dickinson 1996]. Although 96% of individual residents had individual updated care plans, the content of the care plans was poor. In addition, only 17% of those unable to articulate choice had a named independent advocate.

REQUIREMENTS

Ideas on achieving high quality care are largely based on common sense, ethics and human rights. The preservation of autonomy is of prime concern to health care and, additionally, care plans provide a key link in the integration of social and health aspects of care and tackle overlaps between them.

- *Philosophy.* This prime goal should be clearly communicated so that all staff understand its central importance. Care should maintain dignity and self respect, recognise religious and cultural beliefs, and identify nutritional needs as well as special needs due to sensory impairment. Spiritual needs of residents, including those with dementia (and their carers), should be tended, and awareness raised in this regard [Methodist Homes 1997]. Conversation and communication underlie all these issues.

- *Assessment.* There are many aspects to the preservation of autonomy, some of which are shown in (Box 12). This indicates the need for a systematic approach to assessment.

- *Care plans.* Central to the preservation of autonomy is the practice of devising and implementing personalised care plans to meet the needs of residents, supported by a key worker.

4. Preserving autonomy

- *Activities*. Older people in long-term care need something to look forward to day by day and not to be subjected to valueless routines. A range of creative and recreational activities should therefore be available and systematically organised. Responsibility for this would be allocated to an activities organiser who may be part of the home or hospital staff, freelance or employed by an agency such as Age Concern. The identified organiser should be supported by enthusiastic care staff. Activity choices may be facilitated by a pin-board or other display or a news sheet, preferably produced by the residents themselves. Appendix 1 shows some possible activities. Ideally, a recreation hobbies room or studio should be available. Volunteers, including relatives and young people, should be encouraged but need proper induction and supervision. The staff costs of the programme should be part of the budget. Fund-raising by relatives and residents themselves might cover the costs of materials. In some cases the local adult education department will help to establish classes. Music and art therapists could further contribute to these programmes. Involvement in activities is a matter of personal choice; there is no place for coercion. Experience indicates that such programmes may be slow to develop initially but residents' enthusiasm to join gradually becomes infectious.

> **Box 12. Some personal needs in preserving autonomy**
> ❏ Personal goals and attainments
> ❏ Individual waking and bed times
> ❏ Clothing preference
> ❏ Activities preference
> ❏ Food preference
> ❏ Preference as to form of address

- *Exercise*. From a health perspective, exercise should be encouraged for all and especially for those who are immobile. It can have cognitive as well as other psychological benefits in dementia sufferers and others [Stones & Dawe 1993; Fiatarone *et al* 1994; Brill *et al* 1995]. A randomised controlled trial amongst the residents of old people's homes has indicated physiological, functional and psychological benefits [McMurdo & Rennie 1993].

- *Environment*. Aspects of the environment are important in preserving autonomy, particularly by ensuring privacy, independence and personalisation of the individual's space. Some of these elements are shown in Box 13.

> **Box 13. Some personal environmental factors**
> ❏ Bedroom access
> ❏ Personal possessions
> ❏ Personal equipment (eg aids, TV, radio, Walkman, chair)
> ❏ Personal storage and cupboards
> ❏ Variable lighting, heating and ventilation

- *Access to advocacy*. The question of advocates has been the subject of two books [Wertheimer 1993; Dunning 1995], indicating the extent to which interest has developed in this field. Although a recent study of nursing home residents' surrogates showed that they cannot accurately express residents' satisfaction with all areas of nursing home care [Lavizzo-Mourey *et al* 1992], advocacy plays an important role in representing and safeguarding the interests of residents, including those from black and minority ethnic communities.

Clinical effectiveness and clinical guidelines

CARE GUIDELINE

ASSESSMENT

All residents should have a documented assessment on entry, and regularly thereafter, that covers:

- Specific aspects of preserving autonomy
- Identification of opportunities for promoting autonomy

CARE PLAN

All residents should have an implemented personalised care plan that covers:

- The goals of care and the roles of different staff members
- Specific aspects of care:
    - The range of personal needs and preferences
    - Personal clothing
    - Activity programme
    - Respect
    - Communication
    - Choice
- Regular review of the implementation and effectiveness of the plan
- Regular review by a key worker
- Regular review of the need for involvement of an advocate

ENVIRONMENT

All residents should experience an appropriate environment, including:

- Personal environmental needs
- Personal possessions
- Preservation of privacy
- Facilities for recreational and social activities

SPECIALIST ACCESS

All residents should have access to the assistance of an independent advocate.

INFORMATION, INVOLVEMENT AND SATISFACTION

All residents and their relatives should:

- Have clearly communicated information and involvement in the care plan
- Be regularly consulted about the policy, plans, staff development and quality improvement for *preserving autonomy*
- Be satisfied with their care and happy to stay

4. Preserving autonomy

ORGANISATIONAL IMPLICATIONS

COMMITMENT

All long-term care facilities should show commitment to *preserving autonomy* by:

- Having a policy as described below
- Effectively communicating this to all staff on joining, and at regular intervals
- Providing the required resources to put the policy into action, including an activities organiser
- Supporting the policy by staff development and quality improvement

POLICY AND PLANNING

All long-term care facilities should have a written agreed policy to implement the care guidelines that includes:

- A philosophy of *preserving autonomy*
- The role of different staff members and others in working as a team
- The approach to assessment, particularly on entry
- The procedure for devising and implementing a personalised care plan, including detailed contents, review mechanism, onward referral system, and role of the key worker
- Relevant aspects of the environment
- Agreements on access to specialists
- The provision of information to and involvement of residents and relatives, as well as a commitment to satisfaction

STAFF DEVELOPMENT

All long-term care facilities should support the policy by regular staff development activities that:

- Are structured, organised and comprehensive
- Are relevant to all levels of staff
- Cover the range of required knowledge, attitudes, skills (including communication skills) and roles
- Are developed, implemented and evaluated using principles of adult learning

QUALITY IMPROVEMENT

All long-term care facilities should carry out quality improvement activities, such as clinical audit, to achieve high standards in *preserving autonomy*.

5. Promoting urinary continence *(updated)*

RATIONALE

Urinary incontinence is common in long-term care and is associated with reduced quality of life [Grimby *et al* 1993] and unnecessary costs when it can be avoided or prevented. However, urinary incontinence is not an unavoidable consequence of old age. The prevalence of urinary incontinence remains unacceptably high in long-term care facilities with varying figures of 30–53% in nursing homes and 55–80% in long-stay hospital wards [Peet *et al* 1995; RCP 1995]. The average incontinent patient requires about one hour of nursing time daily and this represents 83% of the cost of urinary incontinence; the remaining 13% being laundry and 4% pads and equipment [Borrie & Davidson 1992].

QUALITY OF CARE

The high prevalence of urinary incontinence indicates the need for better care. In a recent audit only half the residents had the cause of their incontinence recorded and a management plan for the treatment. Consultation with a continence advisor had been obtained for 14% of residents with incontinence, even though all facilities had access to continence advisors. Most facilities had a policy for screening off commodes and toilets, monitoring the smell of urine and regularly reviewing methods to promote continence, but few had guidelines for the use of sheath urinals, consent for insertion of catheters and use of prophylactic antibiotics. The CARE scheme evaluation project showed regular toileting to be the most common method of management and drug treatment to be the least used [J Brocklehurst, personal communication]. Findings from a large survey indicated that there was greater emphasis on incontinence management than on continence promotion [Peet *et al* 1996].

REQUIREMENTS

Promoting urinary continence appears daunting because of its prevalence and complexity, but some simple approaches emerge.

- *General.* There needs to be a general understanding that the promotion of urinary continence is a legitimate goal of care. Although urinary incontinence is common it is amenable to a range of interventions.

- *Assessment.* There are standard methods for assessing the nature and severity of urinary incontinence such as the Barthel ADL Index. Impaired mobility and cognitive function remain important predictors

- *Diagnosis.* There is a range of causes of urinary incontinence as shown in Box 14. Identification of the cause will aid management as indicated. Detrusor instability causing urgency and frequency is the most common cause of incontinence in older people [Geirsson *et al* 1993].

- *Care plan.* This should express a holistic management plan and the use of the various approaches to promoting urinary continence. In general, conservative measures should be tried initially; when there are multiple causes the main problem should be tackled first.

- *Environment.* Residents need to be within reach of a toilet, *en suite* facilities or commode; a distance of 12 metres has been suggested. Commodes are often provided for residents with impaired mobility and urinary incontinence. However, disadvantages include lack of privacy, embarrassment, unpleasant smells especially when confined to one room, and the very appearance of a commode [Naylor & Mulley 1993]. *En suite* facilities are therefore preferable to commodes. Toilets should have adequate space and appropriate seats, grab rails and paper dispensers.

- *Containment measures.* Absorbent garments and bed pads may be required while investigations and treatment are underway, or if incontinence is found to be intractable. They require personalised provision. Indwelling catheters and penile sheaths have limited use in this regard.

- *Access.* There should be access to the specialist expertise, investigations and advice of the local continence advisor. Referral should occur when diagnosis is not possible or when initial management over 3 months has failed [RCP 1995].

Box 14. Causes and treatment of urinary incontinence

Cause	Management
Transient	
❏ Any acute disease (by causing weakness and immobility)	Treatment of underlying disease
❏ Urinary infection	Appropriate treatment
❏ Delirium	Treatment of underlying disease
❏ Faecal impaction	Disimpaction and preventive scheme
❏ Medication (diuretics, anticholinergics)	Amend prescription
❏ Atrophic vaginitis	Oestrogen [Fantl *et al* 1994]
❏ Retention of urine	Treatment of underlying cause
❏ Disability	Treatment of health problems, rehabilitation, aids, adaptations
❏ Environmental factors	Adapt environment as required
Established	
❏ Detrusor instability	Bladder retraining, medication
❏ Chronic cerebral disease (eg dementia)	Timed voiding [Colling *et al* 1992; Harke & Richgels 1992; Schnelle *et al* 1993; Burgio *et al* 1994], containment
❏ Genuine stress incontinence	Pelvic floor exercises, electrical treatment, bladder training, devices
❏ Outflow tract obstruction	Medication, surgery
❏ Incomplete emptying	Intermittent self-catheterisation, medication
❏ Spinal cord disease (eg cervical myelopathy)	
❏ Autonomic neuropathy (diabetes)	
❏ Mixed and others	

Clinical effectiveness and clinical guidelines

CARE GUIDELINE

ASSESSMENT

All residents should have a documented assessment on entry, when urinary incontinence occurs and at regular intervals that covers:

- Assessment for the presence and severity of any urinary incontinence using a recognised scale (such as the Barthel ADL Index)
- A clear diagnosis by a specialist of the cause(s) of any urinary incontinence
- Identification of opportunities to promote urinary continence

CARE PLAN

All residents with urinary incontinence should have an implemented personalised care plan that covers:

- The goals of care and the roles of different staff members
- Specific aspects of care:
    - Management of the underlying cause of incontinence
    - Containment measures
- Regular review of the implementation and effectiveness of the plan
- Regular review of the need for referral for expert advice

ENVIRONMENT

All residents with urinary incontinence should be in an environment that helps preserve urinary continence (ensuring privacy by being within 12 metres of a toilet or commode).

SPECIALIST ACCESS

All residents with urinary incontinence should have access to a local expert such as a continence advisor.

INFORMATION, INVOLVEMENT AND SATISFACTION

All residents with urinary incontinence and their relatives should:

- Have clearly communicated information and involvement in the care plan
- Be regularly consulted about the policy, plans, staff development and quality improvement for *promoting urinary continence*
- Be satisfied with their care

ORGANISATIONAL IMPLICATIONS

COMMITMENT

All long-term care facilities should show commitment to *promoting urinary continence* by:

- Having a policy as described below
- Effectively communicating this to all staff on joining, and at regular intervals
- Providing the required resources to put the policy into action
- Supporting the policy by staff development and quality improvement

POLICY AND PLANNING

All long-term care facilities should have a written agreed policy to implement the care guidelines that includes:

- A philosophy of *promoting urinary continence*
- The role of different staff members and others in working as a team
- Background information on the nature and causes of incontinence
- The approach to assessment
- Management (including use of catheters)
- The procedure for devising and implementing a personalised care plan, including detailed contents, review mechanism and onward referral system
- Relevant aspects of the environment
- Agreements on access to specialists
- The provision of information to and involvement of residents and relatives, as well as a commitment to satisfaction

STAFF DEVELOPMENT

All long-term care facilities should support the policy by regular staff development activities that:

- Are structured, organised and comprehensive
- Are relevant to all levels of staff
- Cover the range of required knowledge, attitudes, skills and roles
- Are developed, implemented and evaluated using principles of adult learning

QUALITY IMPROVEMENT

All long-term care facilities should carry out quality improvement activities, such as clinical audit, to achieve high standards in *promoting urinary continence*.

6. *Promoting faecal continence* (updated)

RATIONALE

Faecal incontinence is distressing and unpleasant for all concerned. Problems range from soiling of underclothes to unsocial behaviour such as storing and smearing of faeces. Staff training is important [Colling *et al* 1992], and equally important is the maintenance of residents' dignity and privacy when managing incontinence.

QUALITY OF CARE

The CARE scheme evaluation project showed that, although a treatment plan was written for 64% of incontinent patients, the cause of the faecal incontinence was recorded in only 43%. The most frequent interventions used were regular toileting and regular laxatives. There was an apparent relationship between the frequency of the use of laxatives and the prevalence of faecal incontinence.

REQUIREMENTS

These have been reviewed in a recent report [Royal College of Physicians 1995].

- *General.* An appropriate dictum would be that 'in most cases it is treatable and preventable once a diagnosis has been made' [RCP 1995].

- *Assessment.* As for urinary incontinence, assessment of the nature, severity and underlying cause of faecal incontinence is mandatory.

- *Care plan.* This has the same role as in promoting urinary continence. In general, careful observation (with charting) and patience are required for success. Clinical guidelines for the management of faecal incontinence in primary care have been derived from a consensus conference [Button *et al* 1998]. A recent study indicates that prompted voiding for urinary incontinence has no overall effect on faecal incontinence unless urinary incontinence responds to this intervention [Ouslander *et al* 1996]. One novel procedure reported is the effect of digital stimulation to activate the spinal reflex to overcome constipation [Munchiando & Kendall 1993]. This has been shown to be effective in people with stroke but its acceptability may be limited.

- *Environment.* As for urinary continence.

- *Diagnosis.* Identification of the common causes (ie constipation/faecal impaction, neurogenic incontinence, colorectal disease, diarrhoea, anal sphincter defects, disability) will lead to appropriate treatment (Box 15).

- *Access.* As for urinary continence. Indications for rectal examination and names of staff permitted to undertake this should be clear [Royal College of Nursing 1995].

6. Promoting faecal continence

Box 15. Causes and treatment of faecal incontinence

Cause	Management
❑ Faecal impaction	Empty rectum and colon with daily enemas; prevent recurrence – diet, fluids, exercise, bowel emptying triggered by suppositories [Davies *et al* 1986]
❑ Colorectal disease	Treat underlying disease
❑ Medication (laxatives, magnesium-containing antacids)	Withdraw medication and note effect
❑ Uninhibited defaecation (cognitive impairment or neurogenic)	Prompted bowel programme as for faecal impaction. Or constipating regime with twice weekly enemas for uninhibited defaecation
❑ Mixed and others	

Clinical effectiveness and clinical guidelines

CARE GUIDELINE

ASSESSMENT

All residents should have a documented assessment for the promotion of faecal continence on entry, when faecal incontinence occurs and at regular intervals that covers:

- Assessment of severity and nature of any faecal incontinence using a recognised scale (such as the Barthel ADL Index)
- A clear diagnosis by a specialist of the cause(s) of any faecal incontinence
- Identification of opportunities to promote faecal continence

CARE PLAN

All residents with faecal incontinence should have an implemented personalised care plan that covers:

- The goals of care and the roles of different staff members
- Specific aspects of care:
    - Management of the underlying cause of incontinence
    - Diet and fluid intake
    - Medication
    - Promotion of physical activity
    - Use of laxatives, enemas, suppositories
    - Prevention of constipation
- Regular review of the implementation and effectiveness of the plan
- Regular review of the need for referral for expert advice

ENVIRONMENT

All residents with faecal incontinence should be in an environment that helps preserve faecal continence (being within 12 metres of a toilet or commode which is private, warm and comfortable).

SPECIALIST ACCESS

All residents with faecal incontinence should have access to a local expert such as a continence advisor.

INFORMATION, INVOLVEMENT AND SATISFACTION

All residents with faecal incontinence and their relatives should:

- Have clearly communicated information and involvement in the care plan
- Be regularly consulted about the policy, plans, staff development and quality improvement for *promoting faecal continence*
- Be satisfied with their care

6. Promoting faecal continence

ORGANISATIONAL IMPLICATIONS

COMMITMENT

All long-term care facilities should show commitment to *promoting faecal continence* by:

- Having a policy as described below
- Effectively communicating this to all staff on joining, and at regular intervals
- Providing the required resources to put the policy into action
- Supporting the policy by staff development and quality improvement

POLICY AND PLANNING

All long-term care facilities should have a written agreed policy to implement the care guidelines that includes:

- A philosophy of *promoting faecal continence*
- Background information on the nature and cause of incontinence
- The role of different staff members and others in working as a team
- The approach to assessment
- Management (including the use of laxatives, enemas, suppositories, and general measures such as maintaining fluid intake and promoting mobility)
- The procedure for devising and implementing a personalised care plan, including detailed contents, review mechanism and onward referral system
- Indicators for rectal examination and naming of staff permitted to carry this out
- Relevant aspects of the environment
- Agreements on access to specialists
- The provision of information to and involvement of residents and relatives, as well as a commitment to satisfaction

STAFF DEVELOPMENT

All long-term care facilities should support the policy by regular staff development activities that:

- Are structured, organised and comprehensive
- Are relevant to all levels of staff
- Cover the range of required knowledge, attitudes, skills and roles
- Are developed, implemented and evaluated using principles of adult learning

QUALITY IMPROVEMENT

All long-term care facilities should carry out quality improvement activities, such as clinical audit, to achieve high standards in *promoting faecal continence*.

7. Optimising medication *(updated)*

RATIONALE

High levels of prescribing are a common feature of long-term care affecting most residents who frequently take multiple medication [Lindley *et al* 1992], and up to half may be taking sedatives [Hepple *et al* 1989]. The overuse of inappropriate medication [Gilbert *et al* 1993] is a waste of resources and it may lead to medication induced adverse events, particularly amongst frail older people. On the other hand, the underuse of appropriate medication, such as antidepressants, may deprive older people of effective treatment. Attention has been drawn to these in a recent report [RCP 1997].

QUALITY OF CARE

Standards of medication use in long-term care are thought to be poor. As day to day management of medical conditions (especially incontinence and wounds) is delegated to caring staff, medication reviews principally occur when carers (care staff, family, friends) have noticed side effects, or when the resident's list of medicines is extensive [Williams & Betley 1995]. This is supported by research findings in the USA [Beers *et al* 1991; Beers 1997].

REQUIREMENTS

Pathways to optimising medication are based on the fundamental principles of clinical pharmacology and good prescribing practice rather than on randomised controlled trials. These have been recently reviewed in detail [RCP 1997].

- *General.* The expected goal should be to use the appropriate medication but in minimum doses.

- *Regular medication review.* This is the cornerstone of long-term prescribing. It can be done in a systematic fashion to ensure that each medicine prescribed is appropriate (dose, frequency, route of administration) to the health needs of the resident (Box 16). The review could usefully focus on the use of psychotropic medication and on polypharmacy (ie the various medicines prescribed and their apparent appropriateness and possible interactions) which requires special attention. Education programmes in nursing homes have been shown to facilitate reduction and withdrawal of antipsychotics [Meador *et al* 1997].

- *Psychotropic medication.* A controlled trial has shown how cognitive function can improve after discontinuation of benzodiazepines [Salzman *et al* 1992]. A randomised controlled trial of a comprehensive educational outreach programme, carried out in nursing homes in the USA, resulted in an overall reduction in the use of psychoactive medication and non-recommended hypnotics [Avorn *et al* 1992; Meador *et al* 1997], and a checklist of inappropriate medication has been developed [Beers *et al* 1991; Beers 1997].

- *Access.* All residents with polypharmacy or prescriptions for psychoactive medication should have access to expert advice from a pharmacist. There should be good liaison with pharmacy services, community pharmacists (where and when available) and the GP. Provided an agreement is signed, health commission pharmacists in some areas are paid to provide a service to residential and nursing homes. They could provide medication review and act in a training role, but more incentives are needed.

7. Optimising medication

Box 16. Review of medication

1. Purpose of pharmaceutical review

Reduction in prescribed medication per resident, improvement in residents' quality of life, and improved communication between residents, carers and prescribers.

2. Effective preparation and negotiation

With all interested parties, including the home owner or manager, GPs, caring staff and the residents themselves; the home team should include a pharmacist.

3. Data collection

Baseline information should include current known diagnoses, medication currently prescribed, additional remedies recommended by carers or purchased by patients, and the pattern of medication (as not all medicines are administered in accordance with prescriber's instructions).

4. Pharmaceutical review

Pharmacists may be clinically involved in the residential care setting, and community pharmacists are encouraged to undertake monthly medication reviews for every resident, bringing any anomalies to the attention of the GP. Any recommendations must be clear and specific, soundly based on fact, referenced where possible, and accompanied by suggestions for alternatives.

Clinical effectiveness and clinical guidelines

CARE GUIDELINE

ASSESSMENT

All residents should have a documented assessment that covers:

- Identification of prescriptions for psychoactive drugs, and assessment of their appropriateness
- Identification of polypharmacy,* and assessment of its appropriateness
- Identification of opportunities to optimise medication with non-drug treatments

CARE PLAN

All residents with polypharmacy and/or the use of psychoactive drugs should have an implemented personalised care plan that covers:

- The goals of care and the roles of different staff members
- Specific aspects of care:

    Identification of purpose of all prescriptions

    Minimising the number of drugs

    Simplifying regimes

    Minimising the use of psychoactive drugs

- Regular review of the implementation and effectiveness of the plan
- Regular review of the need for onward referral for expert advice, including liaison between the general practitioner and the pharmacist

SPECIALIST ACCESS

All residents with polypharmacy or prescriptions for psychoactive medication should have access to expert advice both from a pharmacist and from other specialists (eg a psychiatrist).

INFORMATION, INVOLVEMENT AND SATISFACTION

All residents receiving medication and their relatives should:

- Have clearly communicated information and involvement in the care plan
- Be regularly consulted about the policy, plans, staff development and quality improvement for *optimising medication*
- Be satisfied with their care

---

* The term 'polypharmacy' relates to the number of drugs prescribed. A definite number cannot be stated but it depends on the apparent appropriateness of the various drugs and their possible interactions.

7. Optimising medication

ORGANISATIONAL IMPLICATIONS

COMMITMENT

All long-term care facilities should show commitment to *optimising medication* by:

- Having a policy as described below
- Effectively communicating this to all staff on joining, and at regular intervals
- Providing the required resources to put the policy into action
- Supporting the policy by staff development and quality improvement

POLICY AND PLANNING

All long-term care facilities should have a written agreed policy to implement the care guidelines that includes:

- A philosophy of *optimising medication*
- Background information
- The role of different staff members and others in working as a team
- The approach to assessment.
- The procedure for devising and implementing a personalised care plan, including detailed contents, review mechanism and onward referral system
- Relevant aspects of the environment
- Agreements on access to specialists
- The provision of information to and involvement of residents and relatives, as well as a commitment to satisfaction

STAFF DEVELOPMENT

All long-term care facilities should support the policy by regular staff development activities that:

- Are structured, organised and comprehensive
- Are relevant to all levels of staff
- Cover the range of required knowledge, attitudes, skills and roles
- Are developed, implemented and evaluated using principles of adult learning

QUALITY IMPROVEMENT

All long-term care facilities should carry out quality improvement activities, such as clinical audit, to achieve high standards in *optimising medication*.

Clinical effectiveness and clinical guidelines

8. Preventing and managing falls *(updated)*

RATIONALE

Falls in long-term care are common and a public health issue. They are the leading accidental cause of death among older people and a major reason for hospitalisation. Furthermore, falls lead to increased disability and social limitations. Reducing the death rate from accidents in people aged 65 years and older was a Health of the Nation target [Department of Health 1992].

QUALITY OF CARE

Little is known about the present quality of care but it is almost certainly suboptimal. A recent audit study showed that the most common approaches to preventing falls were restraint (41%), sedation (31%), constant supervision of walking (32%) and constant wheelchair use (35%).

REQUIREMENTS

There is increasing evidence concerning the effectiveness of interventions to reduce falls and their consequences. This topic has been recently summarised in a systematic review [NHS Centre for Reviews and Dissemination 1996].

- *General.* Concentrated effort and commitment will be required to tackle this multifactorial challenge.

- *Assessment.* The causes of falls are usually multifactorial. Multiple precipitating factors and risk factors have been identified by a 3-year study. Precipitating factors included: environmental features (50%); physical condition of resident (24%); specific physical activities (7%); and multiple factors (6%) [Fleming & Pendergast 1993]. Risk factors for falls include postural hypotension, use of sedatives, use of more medication, weakness, poor balance, ADL activity, but much of this information is derived from community dwellings subjects [NHS Centre for Reviews and Dissemination 1996]. Other potential risk factors are environmental hazards, lack of exercise, nutritional status, and ageing changes and medical conditions (cognitive impairment, deteriorating vision, nocturia). In a community based study, geriatric syndromes (falls, incontinence, functional dependence) have been attributed to four independent predisposing factors: slow timed chair stands (lower extremity impairment); decreased arm strength (upper extremity impairment); decreased vision and hearing (sensory impairment); and a high anxiety or depression score (affective impairment) [Tinetti *et al* 1995]. Risk factors for recurrent falls in a Finnish study of long-term care residents were: a slow walking speed, a change in living conditions during the previous 2 years, reduced quadriceps strength and the existence of eye disease [Luukinen *et al* 1995]. However, in an American study there were no clear precipitating factors for falls other than severely impaired mobility [Kane *et al* 1995].

- *Multifactorial prevention.* In a randomised controlled trial of a multifactorial intervention among older people in their own homes, the incidence of falls was reduced over one year from 47% to 35% [Rubenstein *et al* 1990]. Intervention to reduce falls amongst long-term care residents should include improving muscle strength and functional status, reducing environmental hazards and identifying and monitoring high risk residents [Rubenstein *et al* 1994, 1996].

8. Preventing and managing falls

- *Exercise.* There is increasingly robust evidence that exercise, particularly balance training, reduces the risk of falling [NHS Centre for Reviews and Dissemination 1996]. Regular exercise is an important preventive measure [Province *et al* 1995] and is feasible within the long-term care setting [Buchner *et al* 1993; Stones & Dawe 1993; Fiatarone *et al* 1994].

- *Psychotropic drugs.* These agents, especially long-acting benzodiazepines, are potent risk factors for falls in older people [Campbell 1991; Trewin *et al* 1992; Yip & Cumming 1994]. In an American study in long-term care the attributable risk among regular psychotropic drug users was 36% [Thapa *et al* 1995]. Others have shown an apparent relationship between the use of antidepressants amongst women and falls in long-term care [Ruthazer & Lipsitz 1993].

- *Shoes.* There are no trials of the role of footwear but shoes should clearly be well fitting.

- *Environment.* Factors that are associated with increased risk of falling are discussed in a recent review [Shroyer 1994] (Box 17).

- *Restraints.* These do not prevent falls. Serious fall-related injuries have been experienced by 5% of unrestrained people compared with 17% of restrained subjects [Tinetti *et al* 1992; Schleenbaker *et al* 1994].

- *Transfers.* Older people are at increased risk of falling when getting out of bed [NHS Centre for Reviews and Dissemination 1996].

- *Hip protectors.* These can dramatically reduce hip fractures [Lauritzen *et al* 1993], but acceptability needs to be explored.

- *Vitamin D/calcium supplementation.* A recent review has shown the potential for preventing fractures by vitamin D/calcium supplementation [NHS Centre for Reviews and Dissemination 1996]. Modelling studies predict a fracture risk reduction of 50% [Reid *et al* 1995], and the numbers needed to treat in order to prevent hip fractures range from 120 in the first year to 12 in the tenth [Gillespie *et al* 1997].

Box 17. Environment and falls

- *Lighting:* low level, low colour contrast
- *Furnishings*: arrangement, low chairs and beds, inappropriate design, poor support
- *Architecture:* absence of safety rails, inconsistent riser height and tread depth of stairs
- *Floor surfaces:* unsecured floor coverings, highly waxed, irregular surface, hard floor surfaces, lack of non-skid surfaces in bathrooms, tubs, kitchens, electrical cords and wires in pathways

Clinical effectiveness and clinical guidelines

CARE GUIDELINE

ASSESSMENT

All residents should have a documented assessment on entry, when a fall occurs and at regular intervals, that covers:

- Assessment of severity and nature of any falls, using documented evidence of the circumstances ('incident form'), symptoms experienced, medication and consequences
- A clear diagnosis of the cause(s) of any falls
- Identification of opportunities to prevent future falls

CARE PLAN

All residents identified as having a risk of falls should have an implemented care plan for prevention covering:

- The goals of care and the roles of different staff members
- Potential risks for falls
- Prevention plan

All residents with a fall should have an implemented personalised care plan that covers the above plus:

- Relevant clinical assessment (inclusive of risk factors)
- Onward referral as required
- Whether the plan has been carried out
- Effectiveness of the plan

ENVIRONMENT

All residents at risk of falling, or who have had a fall, should experience an appropriate environment.

SPECIALIST ACCESS

All residents with recurrent or undiagnosed falls should have access to local specialist advice.

INFORMATION, INVOLVEMENT AND SATISFACTION

All residents with falls and their relatives should:

- Have clearly communicated information and involvement in the care plan
- Be regularly consulted about the policy, plans, staff development and quality improvement for *preventing and managing falls*
- Be satisfied with their care, especially the balance between risk and safety

8. Preventing and managing falls

ORGANISATIONAL IMPLICATIONS

COMMITMENT

All long-term care facilities should show commitment to *preventing and managing falls* by:

- Having a policy as described below
- Effectively communicating this to all staff on joining, and at regular intervals
- Providing the required resources to put the policy into action
- Supporting the policy by staff development and quality improvement

POLICY AND PLANNING

All long-term care facilities should have a written agreed policy to implement the care guidelines that includes:

- A philosophy of *preventing and managing falls*
- The role of different staff members and others in working as a team
- Background information on nature and cause
- The approach to assessment
- Management
- The procedure for devising and implementing a personalised care plan, including detailed contents, review mechanism and onward referral system
- Relevant aspects of the environment
- Agreements on access to local expert advice
- The provision of information to and involvement of residents and relatives, as well as a commitment to satisfaction

STAFF DEVELOPMENT

All long-term care facilities should support the policy by regular staff development activities that:

- Are structured, organised and comprehensive
- Are relevant to all levels of staff
- Cover the range of required knowledge, attitudes, skills and roles
- Are developed, implemented and evaluated using principles of adult learning

QUALITY IMPROVEMENT

All long-term care facilities should carry out quality improvement activities, such as clinical audit, to achieve high standards in *preventing and managing falls.*

Clinical effectiveness and clinical guidelines

9. Preventing and managing pressure sores *(updated)*

RATIONALE

Pressure sores are common in long-term care. In a recent clinical audit, 11% of residents had a grade II, III or IV pressure sore. Pressure sores represent a significant burden of suffering and an unnecessary cost.

QUALITY OF CARE

There is variation in care. In an audit, about a quarter (28%) of residents had no recorded assessment of pressure sore risk using an established instrument. Of those (52%) that were recorded as at risk, 40% were regularly turned, 31% were provided with a special mattress and 24% with a sheepskin.

REQUIREMENTS

There is increasing clarity about the effectiveness of measures to prevent the formation of pressure sores and these have been reviewed for a set of clinical guidelines [Agency for Health Care Policy and Research 1992].

- *Assessment.* The use of risk assessment scales [Norton *et al* 1975; Waterlow 1985] is now widespread, although a recent review has pointed out that few scales have been subjected to full evaluation [NHS Centre for Reviews and Dissemination 1995].

- *Nutritional support.* In a randomised controlled trial comparing two different levels of protein supplementation, higher protein resulted in quicker healing of pressure sores [Breslow & Bergstrom 1994]. Studies of long-term care residents in hospital have shown that they are undernourished [Lipski *et al* 1993; Association of Community Health Councils 1997]. The major reason for patients not getting enough to eat and drink is because they cannot feed themselves as there may be no available help. People who are blind or suffer from dementia or are simply very frail may not even detect the presence of food or drink, and others may be unable to reach or articulate their inability [ACHCEW 1997]. There may therefore be a need to raise awareness and improve training of staff to help meet this concern.

- *Special support surfaces.* The use of different support surfaces has been reviewed recently [NHS Centre for Reviews and Dissemination 1995]. Turning is probably the most expensive intervention so substituting moderately priced alternating pressure mattresses may decrease the overall cost. Less is known about interventions to prevent and treat heel sores. A recent study suggested that an ordinary head pillow was the most effective pressure reducing device [De Keyser *et al* 1994; McNaughton & Brazil 1995].

- *Training.* An educational approach [McNaughton & Brazil 1995] may be of particular relevance in the UK where many care staff are untrained. There are two assessment guides, one for the registered nurse and one for the nursing assistant [King *et al* 1991].

9. Preventing and managing pressure sores

CARE GUIDELINE

ASSESSMENT

All residents should have a documented assessment on entry, when their general condition changes and at regular intervals, that covers:

- Assessment of risk of pressure sore formation using a recognised scale, and identification of opportunities to prevent the development of pressure sores
- Assessment of severity and nature of pressure sores using a recognised grading system
- A clear diagnosis by a specialist of any underlying cause(s) or predisposing factors for any pressure sores

CARE PLAN

All residents identified as being at risk of pressure sore formation should have an implemented personal care plan that includes

- The goals of care and the roles of different staff members
- Skin care: systematic skin inspection, cleansing, avoidance of massage over bony prominences, minimising skin exposure to moisture, proper positioning, turning, protective films and use of creams
- Appropriate mattress/support surface and seating
- Promotion of mobility and activity
- Balanced nutrition
- Regular review of the implementations and effectiveness of the plan

All residents with a pressure sore should have an implemented personal care plan that includes the above plus attention to:

- Dressings
- Pain control
- Regular review of the implementations and effectiveness of the plan

ENVIRONMENT

All residents with a pressure sore should have an appropriate bed and seating support surface.

SPECIALIST ACCESS

All residents with a pressure sore should have access to the advice of a tissue viability expert.

INFORMATION, INVOLVEMENT AND SATISFACTION

All residents with pressure sores or risk of pressure sores and their relatives should:

- Have clearly communicated information and involvement in the care plan
- Be regularly consulted about the policy, plans, staff development and quality improvement for *preventing and managing pressure sores*
- Be satisfied with their care

Clinical effectiveness and clinical guidelines

ORGANISATIONAL IMPLICATIONS

COMMITMENT

All long-term care facilities should show commitment to *preventing and managing pressure sores* by:

- Having a policy as described below
- Effectively communicating this to all staff on joining, and at regular intervals
- Providing the required resources to put the policy into action
- Supporting the policy by staff development and quality improvement

POLICY AND PLANNING

All long-term care facilities should have a written agreed policy to implement the care guidelines that includes:

- A philosophy of *preventing and managing pressure sores*
- The role of different staff members and others in working as a team
- Background and cause
- The approach to assessment
- Management, including treatments to be used
- The procedure for devising and implementing a personalised care plan, including detailed contents, review mechanism and onward referral system
- Relevant aspects of the environment, including local policy for the use of specialised support surfaces and access to well maintained equipment
- Negotiated agreements on access to local expert advice
- The provision of information to and involvement of residents and relatives, as well as a commitment to satisfaction

STAFF DEVELOPMENT

All long-term care facilities should support the policy by regular staff development activities that:

- Are structured, organised and comprehensive
- Are relevant to all levels of staff
- Cover the range of required knowledge, attitudes, skills and roles
- Describe each person's role in *preventing and managing pressure sores*
- Are developed, implemented and evaluated using principles of adult learning

QUALITY IMPROVEMENT

All long-term care facilities should carry out quality improvement activities, such as clinical audit, to achieve high standards in *preventing and managing pressure sores*.

Advice for providers: implementation and outcomes

Providers of long-term care should implement the clinical guidelines in this report. The main mechanism for doing this will be through the use of clinical audit as provided in the revised version of the CARE scheme, and complemented by other approaches such as policy development and staff training. By improving the quality of health care, the quality of life of residents will be enhanced. Experience from other sectors also suggests that providers will reduce their costs when higher quality care is achieved. To put these clinical guidelines in place, five specific actions will be helpful:

- Acting upon the organisational implications of the guidelines
- Establishing a quality improvement procedure such as the CARE scheme
- Training and developing staff
- Developing relationships and agreements with commissioners and others
- Measuring and monitoring outcomes

Acting on the organisational implications

If these are implemented, providers can be confident that high quality care will be delivered. Most of these implications feature the development of local policies and procedures, particularly in relation to care planning.

Establishing a quality improvement scheme

The best framework for evaluating and improving the quality of care is an agreed quality improvement scheme. Key features of such a scheme should be:

- User focused
- Cyclical
- Concentrated on processes of care
- Carried out by and for care staff
- Supported fully by 'top management'
- Enjoyable, constructive and action focused

This specification is fulfilled by the RCP CARE scheme. This provides a ready made set of audits and instructions for staff. Purchasers could show their commitment to quality improvement through clinical audit by monitoring results and recognising the benefit. The revised version of the CARE scheme will include materials that a long-term care facility could use in assembling a portfolio of evidence to show that there was ongoing and meaningful quality improvement. This might be used by commissioners or regulators.

Advice for providers: implementation and outcomes

Developing relationships and agreements with commissioners and others

For some matters, collaboration will be required with other parties such as purchasers of long-term care, registration and inspection officers, the primary health care and community care teams and the local specialist services for the health care of older people and the psychiatry of old age. This may require the development of common approaches to assessments, procedures, training and information management systems. A very important aspect will be establishing routes of communication and access to health care as indicated in the clinical guidelines.

Beginning to tackle outcomes

Experience suggests that a focus on the processes of care is the key to quality improvement. However, there are motives for measuring the outcomes of long-term care. These can be assessed from the different perspectives of the resident, the carer or the service. The specification for any individual outcome measure is daunting, since it must show feasibility, acceptability, validity, reliability and responsiveness. Moreover, a bundle of measures is probably needed to give a rounded picture of success [CASPE 1991].

Residents

From the residents' perspective, the range of impairment, disability and handicap is important, supplemented by measures of quality of life and satisfaction. Assessment of impairments may involve a wide range of measures but we highlight cognitive function and mood. The Barthel ADL Index is the standard way of measuring primary activities of daily living. However, its floor effect (lowest threshold score) may limit use amongst very disabled residents of nursing homes. Its ceiling effect (highest threshold) indicates the need for a measure of secondary ADL, for which there is less consensus.

In relation to handicap, some progress has been made [Harwood *et al* 1994a,b]; it may be appropriate to focus on social functioning. The recommended way of assessing life satisfaction is the anglicised version of the Philadelphia Geriatric Centre Morale Scale, but in nursing home settings alternatives may be more meaningful. Assessing resident satisfaction may be extremely difficult as residents tend to express satisfaction with the care received and are reluctant to criticise. Carers may need to act as proxies for reporting on residents who are cognitively impaired. When eliciting views from residents it is important for interviewers to establish some form of rapport with residents and/or carers to promote freer expression and truer opinion [Challiner *et al* 1996].

Carers

Carers have a crucial role, so outcome measures must be orientated towards them. This might include consideration of satisfaction with service, reduction in strain (as measured by Carer Strain Index [Robinson 1983]) and psychological well-being (using standard measures of anxiety, depression and distress). A guilt scale is currently being developed [Woods & Matthison 1996].

Services

The Multiphasic Environmental Assessment Procedure (MEAP) consists of various sections, and one dimension of the Policy and Program Information (POLIF) section measures availability of services [Timko & Moos 1991]. Job satisfaction by carer staff can be assessed using the short form of the Minnesota Satisfaction Questionnaire [1977], and psychological well-being by the General Health Questionnaire (GHQ) [Goldberg & Hillier 1979].

SECTION 6

Advice for commissioners/purchasers

Commissioners of long-term care have wide ranging responsibilities, not least their regulatory role. The latter is currently under review and indications are that the new approach will fit better with quality improvement. Commissioners play a pivotal role not only in acting on behalf of residents and the local population but also working effectively with providers and in commissioning partnerships [Skea & Lindesay 1996]. The word 'commissioners' disguises the fact that there are a number of different commissioners (purchasers): health authorities have a responsibility to commission services to meet the needs for nursing care of those who qualify for them under the eligibility criteria for listed categories [NHS Executive 1995]; the evolving role of GP fundholders in purchasing long-term care and associated services for their patients will grow; social service commissioners play an important role in the residential care sector; in addition, many individuals and their families act as their own commissioners by funding long-term care privately, with or without the use of insurance products.

Role of registration and regulation

It is argued that regulation and registration are needed to introduce consistency and minimum standards even when there is increasing deregulation. There are many suggestions for enhancing registration and these have been thoroughly considered in the Burgner report [DoH 1996b]. At present NHS wards are not subject to inspection, though in the past the health authority could request an inspection by the Health Advisory Service. A recent study targeted at inspection officers indicates that the quality of care in nursing homes is monitored unevenly or not at all [Arai 1993]. Consequently there is a need to ensure high standards of care and to monitor quality of care in long term settings.

Improving health care in long-term care

Commissioners could have a major impact on enhancing health care in long-term care by reducing the overall long-term care needs and consumption of their population. Simply requiring the implementation of the clinical guidelines in this report or creating incentives for this would have a very useful effect. Commissioners may have a specific role in improving health care input into long-term care by breaking down barriers that currently inhibit the seamless care provision that a patient should receive when transferring from a hospital to a community setting. Commissioners also have a clear opportunity in relation to quality improvement. Clinical audit, which is now carried out throughout the NHS, has been shown to be effective in long-term care and could be fostered using a recognised approach such as the CARE scheme. Perhaps in the future commissioners may become more discerning in the providers they use. A preferred provider status or premium payment could be based on achievement of a standard or accreditation for health care and other aspects of care in long-term care.

Contract specifications

Health and local authorities must establish robust contract specifications and monitor the quality or value for money of the contracts. Service specifications should include:

- Use of a recognised reference guide, such as *Homes are for living in* [Social Services Inspectorate 1989]
- Use of recognised clinical guidelines for health care, such as this report
- Evidence of appropriate staff development
- Evidence of an appropriate quality improvement system such as clinical audit carried out using the CARE scheme
- Staff training as well as development of adequate staff hand-over period

SECTION 7

Research and development needs

Numerous weaknesses in the research base for long-term care have been exposed through the preparation of this report. Some priorities include:

Service provision

- How can the various agencies best work together for most effective quality of care?
- What are the best ways to develop the knowledge, attitude and skills of long-term care staff and others with a role in long-term care?
- What are the advantages and disadvantages of the 'single care home'?
- What is the role and value of teaching nursing homes?
- What cost savings can be achieved by quality improvement in long-term care?
- How can long-term care facilities receive reward and recognition for high quality?
- What are the roles of general practitioners, geriatricians and psychogeriatricians in long-term care?

Residents

- What are the links between common health problems, disability and quality of life in long-term care residents?
- How can the need for interdisciplinary team involvement be identified?

Carers

- What are the positive and negative experiences of carers?
- What support do family carers receive following admission of a relative to care?
- What interventions can be taken to reduce carer guilt?

Specific interventions

- How can the incidence of faecal incontinence be diminished?
- What are the most effective strategies for challenging behaviour?
- What is the best way to prevent depression in long-term care?
- How can rehabilitation potential be realised in long-term care?
- How effective are simple continence promotion regimens, and what underlies success?
- How can health services assist long-term care facilities in preventing injuries from falls?

Conclusion

The issue of long-term care touches the lives of most people in the UK through personal experience or that of a relative or friend. Its future has wide relevance and implications. Foremost is the link between health and quality of life of older people living in long-term care. These clinical guidelines tackle common health issues in long-term care by bringing together a balance of the perspectives of residents and the evidence of clinical effectiveness from research. It is hoped that they will be adopted widely.

The use of these clinical guidelines will bring benefits in three main ways. First, they will lead to improvements in the standard of health care. Second, cost saving can be expected; in individual homes, higher quality health care is likely to lead to reduced costs; across the population, the positive approach to health is aimed at reducing disability. Third, the clear commitment, backed by training, will lead to an improvement in the morale and competence of staff working in long-term care. Ultimately this will be to the benefit of current and future generations of older people.

This report indicates the steps that will need to be taken by the various parties concerned to promote constructive, critical dialogue. The establishment of a common approach to quality improvement will be the most important step. The revised version of the CARE scheme will provide the sound basis for such a development, as it fits the specification of a robust quality improvement system and is effective and acceptable. At the same time, it offers straightforward opportunities for benchmarking, good practice exchange and meaningful accreditation.

It would not have been possible to produce these clinical guidelines without the insights of residents and their families. Their good health should remain a key goal of future long-term care.

APPENDIX 1

Possible activities

Activity & background information	Contact addresses
Art/Handicrafts *Art, painting, flower arranging, modelling* Creativity and social engagement were greater in a group who had weekly sessions discussing works of art compared with a control group who simply engaged in conversation [Wikström *et al* 1992].	■ British Association of Art Therapists, 11a Richmond Road, Brighton, Sussex BN2 3RL. ■ The Arts Council (and regional Arts Council), 14 Great Peter Street, London SW1P 3NQ. Tel: 0171 333 0100.
Literary *Debating, creative writing, poetry and appreciation*	■ British Association of Creative Therapists (BACT), 122 Petersburg Road, Edgeley Road, Stockport, Cheshire SK3 9RB.
Exercise *Exercise classes, games (catching, bowling), Tai Chi Ch'uan, walks* Some forms of training in old age can make a major contribution to quality of life. Even elderly residents of old people's homes can benefit from participation in regular seated exercise and improve their functional capacity [McMurdo & Rennie 1993].	■ Excel 2000, 1A North Street, Sheringham, Norfolk NR26 8LW. Tel: 01263 825670. ■ Extend, 22 Maltings Drive, Wheathampstead, Herts AL4 8QJ. Tel: 01582 832760.
Hobbies *Cookery, gardening, reading, TV* Many materials are available to help disabled people participate [Counsel and Care 1993c, 1995c].	■ Partially Sighted Society, Queen's Road, Doncaster, South Yorkshire DN1 2NX. Tel: 01302 323 132. ■ Horticultural Therapy, Goulds Ground, Vallis Way, Frome, Somerset BA11 3DW. Tel: 01373 464782. ■ Horticulture for All, c/o Thorngrove Centre, Common Mead Lane, Gillingham, Dorset SP8 4RE. Tel: 01747 822242. ■ Royal National Institute for Deaf People, 19–23 Featherstone Street, London EC1Y 8SL. Tel: 0171 296 8000.
Massage and similar therapies Now becoming popular in long-term care [Simington & Laing 1993]. Research shows effects of massage on anxiety levels similar to that of conversation [Fraser & Kerr 1993]. Familiar touch by staff as a comforting gesture is welcomed by many but may be misinterpreted [McCann & McKenna 1993].	■ International Federation of Aromatherapists, Stamford House, 2–4 Chiswick High Road, London W4 1TH. Tel: 0181 742 2605.
Multisensory environment (Snoezelen) Requires a special room with various sensory stimulations (lights, colours, music, essential oils, touch or massage etc).	■ Lesley Anne Wareing. Head Occupational Therapy, Kings Park Community Hospital, Gloucester Road, Boscombe, Bournemouth BH7 6JE. Tel: 01202 303757, ext 6019.

Appendix 1: Possible activities

Activity & background information	Contact addresses
Music & Dance *Including singing, making music, dance, movement, music appreciation* Music and movement may be particularly appropriate for patients with dementia [Lord & Garner 1993]. Music therapy for older patients is particularly promising. It is an effective and inexpensive way to increase alertness and physical vigour while decreasing isolation. Best response can be elicited from music that has meaning and significance to the individual [Rendall 1991].	■ Council for Music in Hospitals, 74 Queens Road, Hersham, Surrey KT12 5LW. Tel: 01932 252809.
Pets With older psychiatric patients companion dogs promoted interaction, mobility and independence [Haughie *et al* 1992]. Benefits of pet therapy in nursing homes extend to volunteers as well [Frances *et al* 1985; Elliot & Milne 1991; Savishinsky 1992].	■ Animal Welfare Trust, Tylers Way, Watford Bypass, Watford, Herts WD2 8HQ. Tel: 0181 950 8215. ■ Pet Health Council (arranges for dogs to visit residential and nursing homes), 4 Bedford Square, London WC1B 3BA. Tel: 0171 631 3795. ■ Society for Companion Animal Studies, 10B Lenny Road, Callander, Scotland FK17 8BA. Tel: 01877 330996.
Religious observance Religion plays an important part in the well-being of older people, including those with dementia [Levin 1994].	■ Christian Council on Ageing, Epworth House, Stuart Street, Derby DE1 2EQ.
Reminiscence *Including discussion of holidays with holiday snaps and sharing of life experiences* Merits of life story books and reminiscence are well known [Myers 1991; Gibson 1994].	■ Age Exchange Theatre Group, 11 Blackheath Village, London SE3 9LA. Tel: 0181 318 9105.
Social interaction inside *Including birthday parties, seasonal celebrations, family visits, friendly visiting schemes and children's visits* Stipulated quiet room for reading, and not watching TV, especially for residents who have to share a bedroom. Visits from children on a well organised basis, such as the 'Magic Me' Project, have proved to be beneficial.	■ Alzheimer's Disease Society, Gordon House, 10 Greencoat Place, London SW1P 1PH. ■ Counsel and Care, Twyman House, 16 Bonny Street, London NW1 9PG. Tel: 0171 485 1550. ■ Relatives Association, 5 Tavistock Place, London WC1H 9SS. Tel: 0171 916 6055. ■ 'Magic Me' Project, Susan Langford, Tower Hamlets, London. Tel: 0181 983 3544.
Social interaction outside *Going to the pub, out for a meal, visiting relatives/friends, going out to social occasions*	■ National Association for Providers of Activities to Older People (NAPA), Marianne Lvov, 124 Sutherland Avenue, London W9 2QP. Tel:0171 286 8855.

APPENDIX 2

Members of the workshops

MANCHESTER WORKSHOP

Professor John Brocklehurst *(Background paper/Report writer)*
Associate Director, Research Unit, Royal College of Physicians

Dr Yvonne Challiner *(Background paper)*
Consultant Physician in Geriatric Medicine, Ramsgate, Kent

Ms Carol Clegg
Project Manager, King's Fund Organisational Audit, London

Mrs Linda Cruttenden *(Background paper)*
Formerly Matron Manager, Royal Surgical Aid Society–AgeCare, Kent

Ms Rohana Darlington
Creative Activities Coordinator, Age Concern East Cheshire

Dr Edward Dickinson *(Background paper/Report writer)*
Acting Director, Research Unit, Royal College of Physicians

Dr Eileen Fairhurst
Senior Lecturer, Care of Elderly People, Manchester Metropolitan University

Dr John Hughes
Manager, Davenham Hall Nursing Home, Cheshire; Registered Nursing Homes Association

Dr David Jolley *(Background paper)*
Consultant in Old Age Psychiatry, Withington Hospital, Manchester

Mrs Leonie Kellaher
Director of Centre for Environmental Studies in Ageing & Faculty Research Director, University of North London

Mr Jim Kennedy
Assistant Chief Inspector, Social Services Inspectorate, Department of Health, London

Mrs Jean Parker *(Background paper)*
Activities Organiser, Department of Geriatric Medicine, Withington Hospital, Manchester

Dr Linda Patterson
Consultant Physician, Rossendale General Hospital, Burnley, Lancashire

Mr Steve Peacock
Senior Assistant Director Community Care, Ealing, Hammersmith and Hounslow Health Agency

Ms Sylvia Quayle
Group Managing Director, Planning and Healthcare Consultancy Contracts Ltd, Shropshire

Dr Isabel Scougel
Consultant Physician, Care of the Elderly, Falkirk and District Royal Infirmary NHS Trust

Mr Jef Smith
General Manager, Counsel and Care, London

Dr Stuart Talbot
Medical Adviser, Salford and Trafford Health Authority

Ms Jane Tyrer *(Background paper)*
Occupational Therapist, Department of Old Age Psychiatry, Withington Hospital, Manchester

Mrs Dorothy White *(Background paper)*
Chairperson, The Relatives Association, London

Appendix 2: Members of the workshops

LONDON WORKSHOP

Ms Sue Benson
Editor, Journal of Dementia Care

Professor John Brocklehurst *(Background paper/Report writer)*
Associate Director, Research Unit, Royal College of Physicians

Dr Julie Clarke *(Background paper)*
Royal College of General Practitioners, Alzheimer's Disease Society Educational Fellow,
University of Newcastle

Mrs Linda Cruttenden
Formerly Matron Manager, Royal Surgical Aid Society–AgeCare, Kent

Dr Edward Dickinson *(Background paper/Report writer)*
Acting Director, Research Unit, Royal College of Physicians

Miss Penny Dodds
Admiral Nursing, Brighton

Mr Peter Dunn
Social Services Inspectorate Community Care and Ageing Group, Department of Health, London

Ms Alison Ewing
Pharmacy Patient Services Manager, Ladywell Hospital, Salford

Mr Michael Hake
Representing the Association of Directors of Social Services, Solihull Metropolitan Borough Council

Dr Marion Hildick-Smith
Chairman, Royal Surgical Aid Society–AgeCare Medical Committee

Capt. Anthony Hutton *(Organiser)*
Formerly General Secretary, Royal Surgical Aid Society–AgeCare, London

Ms Jane John
Director, Care Consortium, Alzheimer's Disease Society

Mr John Keady *(Background paper)*
Lecturer, Department of Nursing, University of Wales, Bangor; Chair of FOCUS Executive

Dr Alastair Macdonald *(Background paper)*
Consultant and Senior Lecturer in the Psychiatry of Old Age,
Mental Health in the Elderly Community Team, Lewisham and Guy's Mental Health Trust, London

Professor Mary Marshall
Director, Dementia Services Development Centre, Stirling University

Ms Liz Matthews
Directorate Manager, Elderly Mental Health Services, Tameside and Glossop Community and Priority
Services NHS Trust; member of RCN FOCUS Executive

Mr David Miller
Manager, Glendon Nursing Home, Eastbourne; representative of the Registered Nursing Homes
Association

Ms Laraine Moffit
Project worker, Christian Council on Ageing, Dementia Project, Newcastle upon Tyne

Ms Jo Moriarty
Researcher, National Institute for Social Work, London

Mrs Pat Ramdhanie
Chairman, RCN SONIRO (Society of Nursing Inspectors and Registration Officers), London

Appendix 2: Members of the workshops

Ms Caroline Reeves
Matron/Manager, St George's Nursing Home, Surrey

Mr Jef Smith
General Manager, Counsel and Care, London

Ms Marlette de Souza *(Co-ordinator)*
Clinical Guidelines Co-ordinator, Research Unit, Royal College of Physicians

Dr Stuart Talbot
Medical Adviser, Salford and Trafford Health Authority

Mr Brian Tanner *(Organiser)*
Homes Secretary, Royal Surgical Aid Society–AgeCare, London

Ms Catriona Thom
Physiotherapist, Health Services for Elderly People, Royal Free Hospital, London

Dr John Wattis *(Background paper)*
Chairman of the Section for Psychiatry of Old Age, Royal College of Psychiatry; Medical Director of Leeds Community and Mental Health NHS Trust; Senior Lecturer in Psychiatry, University of Leeds

Dr John Wedgwood
Chairman, Royal Surgical Aid Society–AgeCare, London

Mrs Dorothy White *(Background paper)*
Chairperson, The Relatives Association, London

Mr David Wigley
Chief Executive, Methodist Homes for the Aged; representing Voluntary Organisations Involved in Care of the Elderly Sector (VOICES)

Mrs Elizabeth Wilson
Occupational Therapist, Welwyn, Hertfordshire

Mrs Elsie Wood
Relative of a person with Alzheimer's disease, Middlesex

Professor Bob Woods
Professor of Clinical Psychology of the Elderly, University of Wales, Bangor

References

Age Concern. *Elderly depression: survey results*. London: Quality Data Preparation & Age Concern, 1996.

Agency for Health Care Policy and Research. *Pressure ulcers in adults: prediction and prevention*. Rockville, Maryland: AHCPR, 1992.

Alfredson BB, Annerstedt L. Staff attitudes and job satisfaction in the care of demented elderly people: group living compared to long-term care. *Journal of Advanced Nursing* 1994;**19**:964–74.

Ames D. Depressive disorders among elderly people in long-term institutional care. *Australian and New Zealand Journal of Psychiatry* 1993;**27**:379–91.

Arai Y. Quality counts. *Health Service Journal* 1993;**103**:33.

Armstron-Esther CA, Brown KD, McAfee JG. Elderly patients: still clean and sitting quietly. *Journal of Advanced Nursing* 1994;**19**:264–71.

Aronson MK, Cox D, Guastadisegni P. Dementia, agitation and care in the nursing home. *Journal of the American Geriatrics Society* 1993;**41**:507–12.

Association of Community Health Councils for England and Wales. *Hungry in Hospital*. London: ACHCEW, 1997.

Avorn J, Soumerai SB, Everitt DE *et al*. A randomised trial of a programme to reduce the use of psychoactive drugs in nursing homes. *New England Journal of Medicine* 1992;**327**:168–73.

Baillon S, Scothern G, Neville P, Boyle A. Factors that contribute to stress in care staff in residential homes for the elderly. *International Journal of Geriatric Psychiatry* 1996;**11**:219–26.

Banerjee S, Shamash K, Macdonald AJD, Mann AH. Randomised controlled trial of effect of intervention by psychogeriatric team on depression in frail elderly people at home. *British Medical Journal* 1996;**313**:1058–61.

Beck C, Modlin T, Heithoff K, Shue V. Exercise as an intervention for behaviour problems. *Geriatric Nursing* 1992; September/October:273–5.

Beers MH. Explicit criteria for determining potentially inappropriate medication use by the elderly: an update. *Archives of Internal Medicine* 1997;**157**:1531–6.

Beers MH, Ouslander JG, Rollingher I *et al*. Explicit criteria for determining inappropriate medication use in nursing homes. Archives of Internal Medicine 1991;**151**:1825–32.

Bender M, Levens V, Goodson C. *Welcoming your clients*. Bicester: Winslow Press, 1996.

Berg L, Buckwalter KC, Chafetz PK *et al*. Special care units for people with dementia. *Journal of the American Geriatrics Society* 1991;**39**:1229–36.

Borrie ME, Davidson HA. Incontinence in institutions: costs and contributing factors. *Canadian Medical Association Journal* 1992;**147**:322–8.

Bowman C. Nursing homes: their demands on primary care. *Geriatric Medicine* 1996; November: 25–6.

Breslow RA, Bergstrom N. Nutritional prediction of pressure ulcers. *Journal of the American Dietetic Association* 1994;**94**:1301–4.

Brill PA, Drimmer AM, Morgan LA *et al*. The feasibility of conducting strength and flexibility programs for elderly nursing home residents with dementia. *Gerontologist* 1995;**35**:263–6.

Brocklehurst J, Dickinson E. Autonomy for elderly people in long-term care. *Age and Ageing* 1996; **25**:329–32.

Buchner DM, Cress ME, Wagner EH *et al*. The Seattle FICSIT/MoveIt study: the effect of exercise on gait and balance in elderly adults. *Journal of the American Geriatrics Society* 1993;**41**:321–5.

Burgener SC, Barton D. Nursing care of cognitively impaired institutionalised elderly. *Journal of Gerontological Nursing* 1991;**17**:37–43.

Burgener S, Jirovec M, Murrell L *et al*. Caregiver and environmental variables related to difficult behaviour in institutionalised demented elderly persons. *Journal of Gerontology* 1992;**47**:242–9.

References

Burgio LD, McCormick KA, Scheve AS et al. The effects of changing prompted voiding schedules in the treatment of incontinence in nursing home residents. *Journal of the American Geriatrics Society* 1994;**42**:315–20.

Buschmann MT, Hollingur LM. Influence of social support and control on depression in the elderly. *Clinical Gerontologist* 1994;**14**:13–28.

Button D, Roe B, Webb C et al. Consensus guidelines for the promotion and management of continence by primary health care teams. *Journal of Advanced Nursing* 1998;**27**:91–9.

Campbell AJ. Drug treatment as a cause of falls in old age: a review of the offending agents. *Drugs and Aging* 1991;**1**:289–302.

CASPE Research/Freeman Outcomes Study. Ed Bardsley M, Coles J. London: CASPE, 1991.

Centre for Policy on Ageing. *A better home life*. London: CPA, 1996.

Challiner Y, Julious S, Watson R, Philp I. Quality of care, quality of life, and the relationship between them in long-term care institutions for the elderly. *International Journal of Geriatric Psychiatry* 1996;**11**:883–8.

Chambers R, Knight F, Campbell. A pilot study of the introduction of audit into nursing homes. *Age and Ageing* 1996;**25**:465–9.

Chartock P, Nevin A, Rzetlelny H, Gilberto P. A mental health training programme in nursing homes. *Gerontologist* 1988;**28**:503–7.

Chester R, Smith J. *Elderly people's sadness*. A study of elderly people with depression. London: Counsel and Care, 1995.

Clark P, Bowling A. Quality of everyday life in long-stay institutions for the elderly: an observational study of long-stay hospital and nursing home care. *Social Science and Medicine* 1990;**30**:1201–10.

Colling J, Ouslander J, Hadley BJ et al. The effects of patterned urge-response toileting (PUT) on urinary incontinence among nursing home residents. *Journal of the American Geriatrics Society* 1992;**40**:135–41.

Counsel and Care. *From home to a home*. London: Counsel and Care, 1992a

Counsel and Care. *What if they hurt themselves?* London: Counsel and Care, 1992b.

Counsel and Care. *The right to take risks*. London: Counsel and Care, 1993a.

Counsel and Care. *People not parcels*. A discussion document to explore the issues surrounding the use of electronic tagging on elderly people in residential care and nursing homes. London: Counsel and Care, 1993b.

Counsel and Care. *Not only bingo*. London: Counsel and Care, 1993c.

Counsel and Care. *Last rights*. London: Counsel and Care, 1995a.

Counsel and Care. *Older people's sadness*. London: Counsel and Care, 1995b.

Counsel and Care. *Leisure, later life and homes*. Ed Clarke A, Hollands J. London: Counsel and Care, 1995c.

Counsel and Care. *Windows to a damaged world*. Ed Clarke A, Hollands J, Smith J. London: Counsel and Care, 1996a.

Counsel and Care. *Home in on quality: 3 – Restraints*. London: Counsel and Care, 1996b.

Davies AD, Snaith PA. The social behaviour of geriatric patients at mealtimes: an observational and an interventional study. *Age and Ageing* 1980;**9**:93–9.

Davies A, Nagelbout MJ, Hoban M, Barnard B. Bowel management: a quality assurance approach to upgrading programs. *Journal of Gerontological Nursing* 1986;**12**:13–7.

De Keyser G. Dejaeger E, De Meyst H, Eders GC. Pressure-reducing effects of heel protectors. *Advances in Wound Care* 1994;**7**:30–2.:

Department of Health. *Health of the Nation*. A strategy for health in England. London: HMSO, 1992.

Department of Health. *Implementing caring for elderly people: the F factor; reasons why some elderly people choose residential care*. London: SSI, DoH, 1994.

References

Department of Health. *Sensory impairment*. London: DoH, 1995.

Department of Health. *In the patient's interest*. Multiprofessional working across organisational boundaries. Report by the Standing Medical and Nursing and Midwifery Advisory Committees (SMNAC). London: DoH, 1996a.

Department of Health. *The regulation and inspection of social services*. London: DoH, 1996b.

Department of Health. *Multiprofessional working and learning: sharing the educational challenge*. London: DoH, 1997.

Dickinson EJ. Long-term care of older people (editorial). *British Medical Journal* 1996;**312**:862–3.

Dickinson EJ, Brocklehurst J. Improving the quality of long-term care for older people: lessons from the CARE scheme. *Quality in Health Care* 1997;**6**:160–4.

Dimond T. Social policy and everyday life in nursing homes: a critical ethnography. *Social Science and Medicine* 1986;**23**:1287–95.

Duncan MT, Morgan DL. Sharing the caring: family care-givers' views of their relationships with nursing home staff. *Gerontologist* 1994;**34**:235–44.

Dunning A. *Citizen advocacy with elderly people*. London: Centre for Policy on Ageing, 1995.

Elliot V, Milne D. Patients' best friend? *Nursing Times* 1991;**87**:34–5.

Elon R. The nursing home medical director role in transition. *Journal of the American Geriatrics Society* 1993;**41**:131–5.

Engle VF, Graney Marshall J. Stability and improvement of health after nursing home admission. *Journal of Gerontology* 1993;**48**:S17–S23.

Evers HK. Care of the elderly sick in the UK. In: *Nursing elderly people*. Ed Redfern S. Edinburgh: Churchill Livingstone, 1991:417–36.

Fantl JA, Cardozo L, McClish DK. Oestrogen therapy in the management of urinary incontinence in postmenopausal women: a meta-analysis. First report of the Hormones and Urogenital Therapy Committee. *Obstetrics and Gynaecology* 1994;**83**:12–8.

Feldt KS, Ryden HB. Aggressive behaviour: evaluating nursing assistants. *Journal of Gerontological Nursing* 1992;**18**:3–12.

Fiatarone MA, O'Neill EF, Ryan ND *et al*. Exercise training and nutritional supplementation for physical frailty in very elderly people. *New England Journal of Medicine* 1994;**330**:1769–75.

Finkel SI, Lyons JS, Anderson RL. A Brief Agitation Rating Scale (BARS) for nursing home elderly. *Journal of the American Geriatrics Society* 1993;**41**:50–2.

Fleming BE, Pendergast DR. Physical condition, activity pattern and environment as factors in falls by adult care facility residents. *Archives of Physical Medicine and Rehabilitation* 1993;**74**:627–30.

Frances G, Turner JT, Johnson SB. Domestic animal visitation as a therapy with adult home residents. *International Journal of Nursing Studies* 1985;**22**:201–6.

Fraser J, Kerr JR. Psychophysiological effects of back massage on elderly institutionalised patients. *Journal of Advanced Nursing* 1993;**18**:238–45.

Friedman R, Gryfe CI, Tal DT, Freedman M. The noisy elderly patient: prevalence, assessment, and response to the antidepressant doxepin. *Journal of Geriatric Psychiatry and Neurology* 1992;**5**:187–91.

Geirsson G, Fall M, Lindstrom S. Subtypes of overactive bladder in old age. *Age and Ageing* 1993;**22**:125–31.

Gerety MB, Williams JW, Mulrow CD *et al*. Performance of case-finding tools for depression in the nursing home: influence of clinical and functional characteristics and selection of optimal threshold scores. *Journal of the American Geriatrics Society* 1994;**42**:1103–9 (GDS).

Gibson F. *Reminiscence and recall: a guide to good practice*. London: Age Concern, 1994.

Gilbert A, Owen N, Innes JM *et al*. Trial of an intervention to reduce chronic benzodiazepine use among residents of aged-care accommodation. *Australian and New Zealand Journal of Medicine* 1993;**23**:343–7.

References

Gillespie WJ, Henry DA, O'Connell DL, Robertson J. *Vitamin D and vitamin D analogues in the prevention of fractures in involutional and post-menopausal osteoporosis.* Cochrane Library. Oxford: Update Software, 1997.

Gilloran AJ, McGlew T, McKee K et al. Measuring the quality of care on psychogeriatric wards. *Journal of Advanced Nursing* 1993;**18**:269–75.

Gilloran A, Robertson A, McGlew T, McKee K. Improving work satisfaction amongst nursing staff and quality of care for elderly persons with dementia: some policy implications. *Ageing and Society* 1995;**15**:375–91.

Gladstone JW. Elderly married persons living in long-term care institutions: a qualitative analysis of feelings. *Ageing and Society* 1995;**15**:493–513.

Godlove C, Dunn G, Wright H. Caring for old people in New York and London: the 'nurses' aide' interviews. *Journal of the Royal Society of Medicine* 1980;**73**:713–23.

Goffman E. On the characteristics of total institutions. In: Cressy DR, ed. *The prison.* New York: Holt, Rinehart & Winston, 1961.

Goldberg DP, Hillier VF. A scaled version of the General Health Questionnaire. *Psychological Medicine* 1979;**9**:139–45.

Grimby A, Milson I, Molander U et al. The influence of urinary incontinence on the quality of life of elderly women. *Age and Ageing* 1993;**22**:82–9.

Guaita A, Jones MJD, Uitali S. *Gentlecare: a new prosthetic approach to the care of demented elderly people.* Proceedings of 3rd European Congress of Gerontology, 1995.

Hallberg IR, Norberg A. Nurses' experiences of the strain and their reactions in [sic] the care of severely demented patients. *International Journal of Geriatric Psychiatry* 1995;**10**:757-66.

Harke JM, Richgels K. Barriers to implementing a continence program in nursing homes. *Clinical Nursing Research* 1992;**1**:158–68.

Harnett DS. Psychopharmacologic treatment of depression in the medical setting. *Psychiatric Annals* 1994;**24**:545–51.

Harwood RH, Ebrahim S. Assessing the effectiveness of audit in long-stay hospital care for elderly people. *Age and Ageing* 1994;**23**:287–92.

Harwood RH, Rogers A, Dickinson E, Ebrahin S. Measuring handicap: the London handicap scale, a new outcome measure for chronic disease. *Quality in Health Care* 1994a;**3**:11–6.

Harwood RH, Jitapunkul S, Dickinson E, Ebrahim S. Measuring handicap: motives, methods and a model. *Quality in Health Care* 1994b;**3**:53–7.

Haughie E, Milne D, Elliot V. An evaluation of companion dogs with elderly psychiatric patients. *Behavioural Psychotherapy* 1992;**20**:367–72.

Hepple J, Bowler J, Bowman CE. A survey of private nursing home residents in Weston-Super-Mare. *Age and Ageing* 1989;**18**:61–3.

Hermann N, Mittmann N, Silver IL et al. A validation study of the geriatric depression scale short form. *International Journal of Geriatric Psychiatry* 1996;**11**:457–60.

Heston LL, Garrard J, Makris L et al. Inadequate treatment of depressed nursing home elderly. *Journal of the American Geriatrics Society* 1992;**40**:1117–22.

Hewison A. Nurses' power in interactions with patients. *Journal of Advanced Nursing* 1995;**21**:75–82.

Inouye SK, Van Dyck CH, Alessi CA et al. Clarifying confusion: the confusion assessment method. *Annals of Internal Medicine* 1990;**113**:941-8.

Jones GM, Ely S, Miesen BML. The need for an interdisciplinary care curriculum for professionals working with dementia. In: *Caregiving in dementia: research and applications.* Ed Jones GMM, Miesen BML. London: Routledge, 1992:437–53.

Kane RL, Garrard J, Buchanan JL et al. Improving primary care in nursing homes. *Journal of the American Geriatrics Society* 1991;**39**:359–67.

References

Kane RS, Burns EA, Goodwin JS. Minimal trauma fractures in elderly nursing home residents: the interaction of functional status, trauma, and site of fracture. *Journal of the American Geriatrics Society.* 1995;**43**:156–9.

Katz PR, Karuza J, Counrell SR. Academics and the nursing home. *Clinics in Geriatric Medicine* 1995; **11**:503–13.

Kayser-Jones JS. *Old and alone: care of the aged in the UK and Scotland.* Berkeley: University of California Press, 1981/1990.

Kayser-Jones JS. The impact of the environment on the quality of care in nursing homes: a social-psychological perspective. *Holistic Nursing Practice* 1991;**5**:29–38.

Kihlgren M, Kuremyr D, Norberg A *et al.* Nurse-patient interaction after training in integrity promoting care in a long term ward: analysis of video-recorded morning care sessions. *International Journal of Nursing Studies* 1993;**30**:1–3.

King PA, Longman AJ, Pergrin JV. Educating nursing home staff in lower extremity assessment and care. *Geriatric Nursing* 1991;**12**:297–9.

Kitwood T. Person and process in dementia. *International Journal of Geriatric Psychiatry* 1993;**8**:541–5.

Kitwood T, Bredin K. Towards a theory of dementia care: personhood and well-being. *Journal of the Centre for Policy on Ageing and the British Society of Gerontology* 1992a; **12**: 269–87.

Kitwood T, Bredin K. *Person to person: a guide to the care of those with failing mental powers.* Loughton: Gale Centre Publications, 1992b.

Kitwood T, Woods B. *Training and development strategy for dementia care in residential settings.* Bradford Dementia Group: Royal Surgical Aid Society, 1996.

Kivela S, Lehtomaki E, Kivekas J. Prevalence of depressive symptoms and depression in elderly Finnish home nursing patients and home help clients. *International Journal of Social Psychiatry* 1986;**32**:3–13.

Kuremyr D, Kihlgren M, Norberg A *et al.* Emotional experience, empathy and burnout among staff caring for patients at a collective living unit and nursing home. *Journal of Advanced Nursing* 1994; **19**:670–9.

Laing & Buisson. Market review. In: *Laing review of private healthcare.* London: Laing & Buisson Publishers, 1995.

Lardner R, Nicholson E. *Nurse in service training on a psychiatric unit.* Training Report I. Dementia Services Centre, University of Stirling, 1990.

Lauritzen JB, Petersen MM, Lund B. Effect of external hip protectors on hip fractures. *Lancet* 1993; **341**:11–3.

Lavizzo-Mourey RJ, Zinn J, Taylor L. Ability of surrogates to represent satisfaction of nursing home residents with quality of care. *Journal of the American Geriatrics Society* 1992;**40**:39–47.

Levin JS (ed). *Religion in ageing and health: theoretical foundations and methodological frontiers.* London: International Educational and Professional Publisher Thousand Oaks, 1994.

Lindley CM, Tully MP, Paramsotty V, Tallis R. Inappropriate medication is a major cause of adverse drug reactions in elderly patients. *Age and Ageing* 1992; **21**:294–300.

Lipski PS, Torrance A, Kelly PJ, James OFW. A study of nutritional deficits on long-stay geriatric patients. *Age and Ageing* 1993;**22**:244–55.

Lord TR, Garner JE. Effects of music on Alzheimer's patients. *Perceptual and Motor Skills* 1993;**76**:451–5.

Luukinen H, Koski K, Laippala P, Kivela SL. Risk factors for recurrent falls in the elderly in long-term institutional care. *Public Health* 1995;**109**:57–65.

McCann K, McKenna HP. An examination of touch between nurses and elderly patients in a continuing care setting in Northern Ireland. *Journal of Advanced Nursing* 1993;**18**:838–46.

McCue JD. The naturalness of dying. *Journal of the American Medical Association* 1995;**273**:1039–43.

McGivney SA, Milvihill M, Taylor B. Validating the GDS depression screen in the nursing home. *Journal of the American Geriatrics Society* 1994;**42**:490–2.

References

McGrath AM, Jackson GA. Survey of neuroleptic prescribing in residents of nursing homes in Glasgow. *British Medical Journal* 1996;**312**:611–2.

McMurdo MET, Rennie L. A controlled trial of exercise by residents of old people's homes. *Age and Ageing* 1993;**22**:11–5.

McNaughton V, Brazil K. Wound and skin team: impact on pressure ulcer prevalence in chronic care. *Journal of Gerontological Nursing* 1995;**21**:45–9.

Mann A, Graham N, Ashby D. Psychiatric illness in residential homes for the elderly: survey in one London borough. *Age and Ageing* 1984;**13**:257–65.

Marsland D, Leoussi AS, Norcross P. Disability abated: audio-cassettes for the visually impaired. *Journal of the Royal Society of Health* 1994;**114**:29–32.

Meador KG, Taylor JA, Thapa PB et al. Predictors of antipsychotic withdrawal or dose reduction in a randomised controlled trial of provider education. *Journal of the American Geriatrics Society* 1997;**45**: 207–10

Methodist Homes. *Quality standards manual.* Derby: Methodist Homes for the Aged, 1997.

Miller L. *Validation therapy: the human face of elderly care?* Paper at British Society of Gerontology annual conference, University of Keele, 1995.

Minnesota Satisfaction Questionnaire: a measure of employee job satisfaction (short form). University of Minnesota, 1977.

Moriarty J, Webb S. *Part of their lives: an evaluation of community care arrangements for older people with dementia.* London: National Institute for Social Work, 1997.

Morley JE, Kraenzie D. Causes of weight loss in a community nursing home. *Journal of the American Geriatrics Society* 1994;**42**:583–5.

Morris JN, Haes C, Fries BE et al. Designing the national residential assessment instrument. *Gerontologist* 1990:**30**:293–307.

Munchiando JF, Kendall K. Comparison of effectiveness of two bowel programmes for CVA patients. *Rehabilitation Nursing*, 1993;**18**:168–72.

Murphy E. Quality assurance in residential care (editorial). *International Journal of Geriatric Psychiatry* 1992;**7**:695–7.

Myers KH. *Life story books.* Stirling: Dementia Services Development Centre, 1991.

Nagel J, Cimbolic P, Newlin M. Efficacy of elderly and adolescent volunteer counsellors in a nursing home setting. *Journal of Counselling Psychology* 1988;**35**:81–6.

Naylor JR, Mulley GP. Commodes: inconvenient conveniences. *British Medical Journal* 1993;**307**: 1258–60.

Nelson J. The influence of environmental factors in incidents of disruptive behaviour. *Journal of Gerontological Nursing* 1995;**21**:19–24.

NHS Centre for Reviews and Dissemination. *Effective health care: the prevention and treatment of pressure sores.* Nuffield Institute for Health, University of Leeds; University of York. Churchill Livingstone, 1995.

NHS Centre for Reviews and Dissemination. *Effective health care: preventing falls and subsequent injury in elderly people.* Nuffield Institute for Health, University of Leeds; University of York. Churchill Livingstone, 1996.

NHS Executive. *Responsibilities for meeting continuing care needs.* HSG(95)8. Leeds: NHSE, 1995.

Nolan MR. *Education for change: an evaluation of a teaching programme in five residential homes in Powys.* Bangor: University of Wales, BASE Practice Research Unit, 1992.

Nolan MR, Walker G. *The next best thing to my own home: an evaluation of a sheltered tenant housing scheme in Clwyd.* Bangor: University of Wales, BASE Practice Research Unit, 1993.

Nolan MR, Owens RG, Nolan J. Continuing professional education: identifying the characteristics of an effective system. *Journal of Advanced Nursing* 1995a;**21**:551–60.

Nolan MR, Grant G, Nolan J. Busy doing nothing: activity and interaction levels amongst differing populations of elderly patients. *Journal of Advanced Nursing* 1995b;**22**:528–38.

Norton D, Exton-Smith AN, McLaren R. *An investigation of geriatric nursing problems in hospitals.* National Corporation for Care of Old People. London: Churchill Livingston, 1962 (reprinted 1975).

Nystrom AM, Segerston KM. On sources of powerlessness in nursing home life. *Journal of Advanced Nursing* 1994;**19**:124–33.

Ouslander JG, Simmons S, Schnelle J et al. Effects of prompted voiding on faecal continence among nursing home residents. *Journal of the American Geriatrics Society* 1996;**44**:424–8.

Palmer MH. Nurses' knowledge and belief about continence interests in long-term care. *Journal of Advanced Nursing* 1995;**21**:1065–72.

Parker G, Hadzi-Pavlovic D. Prediction of response to antidepressant medication by a sign-based index of melancholia. *Australian and New Zealand Journal of Psychiatry* 1993;**27**:56–61.

Pearson A, Hocking S, Mott S, Riggs A. Quality of care in nursing homes: from the resident's perspective. *Journal of Advanced Nursing* 1993;**18**:20–4.

Peet SM, Castleden CM, McGrother CW. Prevelence of urinary and faecal incontinence in hospitals and residential nursing homes for older people. *British Medical Journal* 1995;**311**:1063–4.

Peet SM, Castleden CM, McGrother CW, Duffin HM. The management of urinary incontinence in residential and nursing homes for older people. *Age and Ageing* 1996;**25**:139–43.

Podgorski CA, Tariot PN, Blazine L et al. Cross discipline disparities in perceptions of mental disorders in long-term care facility. *Journal of the American Geriatrics Society* 1996;**44**:792–7.

Province MA, Hadley EC, Hornbrook MC et al. The effect of exercise on falls in elderly patients: a preplanned meta-analysis of the FICSIT trials. Frailty and Injuries: Cooperative Studies of Interventive Techniques. *Journal of the American Medical Association* 1995;**273**:1341–7.

Reed J, Bond S. Nurses' assessment of elderly patients in hospital. *International Journal of Nursing Studies* 1991;**13**:418–9.

Reid IR, Ames RW, Evans MC et al. Long term effects of calcium supplementation on bone loss and fractures in postmenopausal women: a randomised controlled trial. American Journal of Medicine 1995;**98**:331–5.

Rendall T. Music not only has charms to soothe but also to aid elderly in coping with various disabilities. *Journal of the American Medical Association* 1991;**266**:1323, 1324, 1329.

Ritchie K, Ledésert B. The families of the institutionalised dementing elderly: a preliminary study of stress in a French caregiver population. *International Journal of Geriatric Psychiatry* 1992;**7**:5–14.

Robertson A, Gilloran A, McGlew T et al. Relationship between job satisfaction and quality of care. *International Journal of Geriatric Psychiatry* 1995;**10**:575–4.

Robinson BC. Validation of a caregiver strain index. *Journal of Gerontology* 1983;**38**:344–8.

Rosenthal CJ, Sulman J, Marshall VW. Depressive symptoms in family caregivers of long-stay patients. *Gerontologist* 1993;**33**:249–57.

Rovner BW, German PS, Broadhead J et al. The prevalence and management of dementia and other psychiatric disorders in nursing homes. *International Psychogeriatrics* 1990; **147**:299–302.

Rovner BW, German PS, Brant LJ et al. Depression and mortality in nursing homes. *Journal of the American Medical Association* 1991;**265**:993–6.

Rovner BW, Steele CD, Schmuely DAW, Folstein MT. A randomised trial of dementia care in nursing homes. *Journal of the American Geriatrics Society* 1996;**44**:7–13.

Royal College of Nursing Continence Care Forum. *Digital rectal examination and manual evacuation of faeces*. London: RCN, 1995.

Royal College of Physicians and the British Geriatrics Society. *High quality long-term care for elderly people*. London: RCP, 1992a.

References

Royal College of Physicians and the British Geriatrics Society. *Standardised assessment scales for elderly people*. London: RCP, 1992b.

Royal College of Physicians. *The CARE scheme (Continuous Assessment Review and Evaluation): clinical audit of long-term care of elderly people*. London: RCP, 1992c.

Royal College of Physicians. *Incontinence: causes, management and provision of services*. London: RCP, 1995.

Royal College of Physicians. *Medication for older people*. London: RCP, 1997.

Royal College of Psychiatrists. *Depression in the elderly*. London: RCPsych, 1996.

Rubenstein LZ, Robbins AS, Josephson KR *et al*. The value of assessing falls in an elderly population: a randomised clinical trial. *Annals of Internal Medicine* 1990;**113**:308–16.

Rubenstein LZ, Josephson KR, Robbins AS. Falls in the nursing home. *Annals of Internal Medicine* 1994;**121**:442–51.

Rubenstein LZ, Josephson KR, Osterweil D. Falls and fall prevention in the nursing home. *Clinics in Geriatric Medicine* 1996;**12**:881–902.

Ruthazer R, Lipsitz LA. Antidepressants and falls among elderly people in long-term care. *American Journal of Public Health* 1993;**83**:746–9.

Salzman C, Fisher J, Nobel K *et al*. Cognitive improvement following benzodiazepine discontinuation in elderly nursing home residents. *International Journal of Geriatric Psychiatry* 1992;**7**:89–93.

Savishinsky JS. Intimacy, domesticity and pet therapy with the elderly: expectations and experiences among nursing home volunteers. *Social Science and Medicine* 1992;**34**:1325–34.

Schleenbaker RE, McDowell SM, Moore RW *et al*. Restraint use and inpatient rehabilitation: incidence, predictors, and implications. *Archives of Physical Medicine and Rehabilitation* 1994;**75**:427–30.

Schneider J, Mann A, Mozley C *et al*. *Residential care for elderly people: policy implications from an exploratory study*. Discussion Paper 1251, Canterbury: Personal Social Services Research Unit, 1997.

Schnelle JF, Ouslander JG, Simmons SF *et al*. The night-time environment, incontinence care, and sleep disruption in nursing homes. *Journal of the American Geriatrics Society* 1993;**41**:910–4.

Scott PA. Care, attention and imaginative identification in nursing practice. *Journal of Advanced Nursing* 1995;**21**:1196–200.

Shroyer JL. Recommendations for environmental design research correlating falls and the physical environment. *Experimental Ageing Research* 1994;**20**:303–9.

Simington JA, Laing GP. Effects of therapeutic touch on anxiety in institutionalised elderly. *Clinical Nursing Research* 1993;**2**:438–50.

Simon RI. Silent suicide in the elderly. *Bulletin of the American Academy of Psychiatry and the Law* 1989;**17**:83–95.

Skea D, Lindesay J. An evaluation of two models of long term residential care for elderly people with dementia. *International Journal of Geriatric Psychiatry* 1996;**11**:233–41.

Social Services Inspectorate, Department of Health. *Homes are for living in*. London: HMSO, 1989.

State University of New York. *Guide for the Uniform Data Set for medical rehabilitation* (Adult FIM), version 4.0. Buffalo: State University of New York, 1993.

Stephens MAP, Kinney JM, Ogrocki PK. Stressors and well-being among caregivers to elderly adults with dementia: the in-home versus nursing home experience. *Gerontologist* 1991;**31**:217–23.

Stones MJ, Dawe D. Acute exercise facilitates semantically cued memory in nursing home residents. *Journal of the American Geriatrics Society* 1993;**41**:531–4.

Stuck AE, Siu AL, Wieland GD *et al*. Comprehensive geriatric assessment: a meta-analysis of controlled trials. *Lancet* 1993:**342**:1032–6.

Sturgess I, Rudd AG, Shilling J. Unrecognised visual problems amongst residents of part III homes. *Age and Ageing* 1994;**23**:54–6.

References

Sumaya-Smith I. Care-giver/resident relationships: surrogate family bonds and surrogate grieving in a skilled nursing facility. *Journal of Advanced Nursing* 1995;**21**:447–51.

Sunderland T, Silver MA. Neuroleptics in the treatment of dementia. *International Journal of Geriatric Psychiatry* 1988;**3**:79–88.

Thapa PB, Gideon P, Fought RL, Ray WA. Psychotropic drugs and risk of recurrent falls in ambulatory nursing home residents. *American Journal of Epidemiology* 1995;**142**:202–11.

Timko C, Moos RH. A typology of social climates in group residential facilities for older people. *Journal of Gerontology* 1991;**46**:5160–9.

Tinetti ME, Lin WL, Ginter SF. Mechanical restraint use and fall related injuries among residents of skilled nursing facilities. *Annals of Internal Medicine* 1992;**116**:369–74.

Tinetti ME, Inouye SK, Gill TM, Doucette JT. Shared risk factors for falls, incontinence, and functional dependence: Unifying the approach to geriatric syndromes. *Journal of the American Medical Association* 1995;**273**:1348–53.

Tolson D, McIntosh J. Hearing impairment in elderly hospital residents. *British Journal of Nursing* 1992; **1**:705–10.

Townsend P. *The last refuge: a survey of residential institutions and homes for the aged*. London: Routledge, 1962.

Trewin VF, Lawrence CJ, Veitch GB. An investigation of the association of benzodiazepine and other hypnotics with the incidence of falls in the elderly. *Journal of Clinical Pharmacy and Therapeutics* 1992; **17**:129–33.

Turoff M. The design of a policy Delphi. *Technological Forecasting and Social change* 1970;**2**:149–71.

Waterlow J. A risk assessment card. *Nursing Times* 1985;**81**:48–55.

Waters K. Getting dressed in the morning: styles of staff/patients interaction on rehabilitation hospital wards for elderly people. *Journal of Advanced Nursing* 1994;**19**:239–48.

Webber C. Training staff to care for patients with Alzheimer's Disease. In: *Carers, professionals and Alzheimer's disease*. Ed O'Neill D. Proceeding of 5th Alzheimer's Disease International Conference. London: John Libbey, 1991.

Webster SGP. In continuing care. *Age and Ageing* 1994;**23**:S36–S38.

Wells TJ. *Problems in geriatric nursing*. Edinburgh: Churchill Livingstone, 1980.

Wertheimer A. *Citizen advocacy and elderly people*. London: Centre for Policy on Ageing, 1993.

Weyerer S, Hafner H, Mann AH et al. Prevalence and course of depression among elderly residential home admissions in Mannheim and Camden, London. *International Psychogeriatrics* 1995;**7**:479–93.

White D. *On being the relative of someone in a home*. London: Relatives Association, 1994.

Wikström BM, Theorell T, Sandstöm S. Psychophysiological effects of stimulation with pictures of works of art in old age. *International Journal of Psychosomatics* 1992;**39**:68–75.

Williams B, Betley C. Inappropriate use of nonpsychotic medications in nursing homes. *Journal of the American Geriatrics Society* 1995;**43**:513–9.

Woods R, Matthison G. *A postal survey of members of the Relatives Association having relatives/friends in residential care*. London: Relatives Association, 1996.

Yip YB, Cumming RG. The association between medication and falls in Australian nursing home residents. *Medical Journal of Australia* 1994;**160**:14–8.

Further reading

SSI (Social Services Inspectorate, Department of Health). *Guidance on standards for residential homes for older people.* HMSO, 1990.

SSI. *Guidance on standards for residential homes for people with a physical disability.* HMSO, 1990.

SSI. *Guidance on standards for residential care needs of people with specific mental health needs.* HMSO, 1992.

SSI. *Guidance on standards for the residential care needs of people with learning disabilities/mental handicap.* HMSO, 1992.

SSI. *Standards for residential care of elderly people with mental disorders.* HMSO, 1993.

SSI. *Responding to residents.* HMSO, 1996.

Relatives' views. Relatives Association, 1993.

'I have come to visit my wife'. Relatives Association, 1996.

Enhancing the role of relatives and residents. Relatives Association, 1996.

Being the relative of somebody in a home. Relatives Association, 1996.

Setting up relatives groups in homes. Relatives Association, 1996.

A relative's perspective. Relatives Association, 1996.

Joint guidelines for the use of medicines in residential homes. Royal Pharmaceutical Society & Age Concern, 1989.

Meeting the costs of continuing care: report and recommendations. York: York Publishing Services, Joseph Rowntree Foundation, 1997. Tel: 01904 431213.

Meeting the costs of continuing care: public views and perceptions. Ed. Diba R. York: York Publishing Services, Joseph Rowntree Foundation, 1997.

Royal College of General Practitioners. *Teamwork in primary care: a policy statement.* London: RCGP, 1992.

Secretaries of State. *Social services achievement and challenge.* London: HMSO, 1997.

Age Concern. *Dementia care.* A handbook for use in residential and day care. Ed. Chapman A, Marshall M, Jacques A. London: Age Concern, 1994.